CURING U.S. HEALTH CARE ILLS

by Bert Seidman

NPA Committee on New American Realities

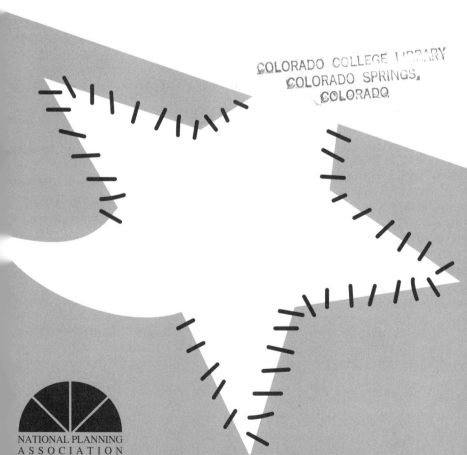

NATIONAL PLANNING
ASSOCIATION

CURING U.S. HEALTH CARE ILLS

NAR Report #6
NPA Report #252

Price $12.00

ISBN 0-89068-108-2
Library of Congress
Catalog Card Number 91-62325

Printed in the United States of America

Contents

Curing U.S. Health Care Ills
by Bert Seidman

Charts

Table

Preface

By the Chair of the Committee on New American Realities

One of the major issues confronting the nation is the crisis in health care and its effects on the American people and our economy. To learn more about the U.S. as well as foreign health care systems and the proposals for changes in the way that health care is financed and delivered in this country, the National Planning Association's Committee on New American Realities held a series of meetings to which we invited outstanding experts in the field. These discussions made clear the gravity of the health care problems facing the nation: the U.S. system is structurally flawed and in crisis; health care costs are out of control; access is difficult for tens of millions; and serious problems continue in the quality and efficiency of much of America's medical care.

These conclusions convinced NAR Committee members of the need for fundamental reorganization of important features of the current health care system. We asked Bert Seidman — who held major health care responsibilities with the AFL-CIO from 1966 to 1990 and served on many public and private advisory bodies — to prepare a report examining the nation's most important health care problems, the proposals for dealing with them, and the solutions that the NAR might consider to help cure the current system's major defects.

The members of the Committee are deeply concerned that although the nation spends $2 billion a day on health care, there are 30-40 million Americans without any health insurance and at least as many with health care coverage that is inadequate to meet their needs. For several years, health insurance premiums have been increasing in double digits, and there is no letup in sight. Most American business and labor leaders see the high cost of health care as a major factor in undermining the competitiveness of American products and services.

In response to this situation, business, labor and health care professionals are examining ways to control costs, provide equality of access and ensure quality services. After a decade of trench warfare over health care costs and cost shifting, the combatants — hospitals, doctors, nurses, insurers, employers, employees, government officials, politicians, and patients — have a sense of winning some battles, but losing the war.

Clearly the defects of the U.S. health care system and the steps that can be taken to correct them are not just a concern of government. With the

vii

stakes so great, private parties — physician and hospital groups, employers, unions, and others affected by the high costs of health care and the gaps in access — must become involved in seeking solutions and offering recommendations.

Remarkable consensus has developed in recent years concerning the defects in the U.S. health care system. The major deficiencies include:
• excessive health care costs;
• no coverage for 31-40 million people;
• the need for quality improvement;
• international competitiveness hampered by health care inflation; and
• inadequate long-term care.

The Committee has examined health care systems in other countries and proposals for reforming health care in America. Although we have not developed a detailed proposal, as representatives of business, labor, agriculture, and academia, we have reached a consensus on the fundamental goals that we regard as essential to the nation's health care system:
• universal coverage;
• comprehensive benefits;
• built-in cost controls;
• improved quality of care;
• a broad range of long-term care services;
• affordable, adequate and equitable financing;
• a favorable impact on U.S. competitiveness; and
• compatibility with American traditions, principles and institutions.

All Committee members do not agree with every point raised in this study, nor will they cease their efforts to find solutions individually and in other forums. They do, however, believe Mr. Seidman has done a most useful job of analyzing the problem and the various approaches to a solution, and they recommend this study to a wider audience as one that will contribute to informed discussion of the issue.

The members of the Committee — as individuals and in the National Planning Association and other organizations — intend to continue to concentrate on the critical problems that the United States faces in health care. The goal of the Committee is to achieve an affordable quality health care system for all Americans.

Charles R. Lee
President and Chief Operating Officer,
GTE Corporation

Executive Summary
Curing U.S. Health Care Ills
by Bert Seidman

America's health care system is in deep trouble, and most Americans are dissatisfied with it.

This pervasive dissatisfaction is not surprising since the United States has the most expensive health care system in the industrialized world, and these spiraling costs are jeopardizing the coverage of the majority of Americans. The latest figures indicate that in 1990 the nation spent an all-time high of 12.2 percent of its gross national product for health care. Health care inflation is unbridled, and there is no end in sight. Yet, except for South Africa, the United States is the only industrialized country with a significant proportion of its population lacking health care coverage.

The demand for health care reform is widespread and insistent. Poll after poll has demonstrated that the American people want fundamental reform of the health care system and they are ready for major change. This is indeed the time for action.

Perceptions about Health Care

Employers have seen expenditures for health care for their employees and families rise unrelentingly over a long period of time. Moreover, the efforts of many firms to restrain health care costs have had little or no effect. Ever mounting health care costs have weakened U.S. competitiveness in markets both at home and abroad.

Leaders of American labor have concluded that the employment-based health care system in the United States that provides health care coverage for most American workers may be collapsing. Many workers, union and nonunion, have seen long-established health care coverage sharply reduced.

The federal government has sought to introduce cost controls in its programs, especially Medicare which provides health care for the elderly and the severely disabled. However, federal health care costs continue to rise rapidly.

Many states face fiscal crises to which rapidly escalating health care costs have largely contributed. For most states, Medicaid costs have become one of their largest spending categories, and they have had to reduce their spending for nonhealth programs to meet their Medicaid obligations.

At least 31 million Americans and perhaps as many as 40 million lack health care coverage. In addition, tens of millions have inadequate coverage.

Technological medical marvels now permit people to be kept alive at enormous expense and often in great pain and discomfort. The sentiment is increasing that prolonging life artificially is unnecessarily costly, ethically wrong and frequently cruel.

Very few Americans have any kind of coverage for long-term health care — either home or nursing home care. With the aging population, the need for long-term care is rapidly expanding. The largest long-term U.S. care program is Medicaid, a welfare program that requires middle-income patients to become paupers to obtain its assistance.

A Consensus about What Is Wrong with U.S. Health Care

In recent years, a remarkable consensus has developed about what is wrong with the nation's health care system. The main conclusions are that:
1. health care costs are excessive and for many years have been rising far faster than the overall inflation rate;
2. depending on estimation methods, 31 million to 40 million people have no health care coverage and at least as many have inadequate coverage;
3. in important respects, quality of care is unsatisfactory and measures to assess it, the only basis on which improvements can be effected, are in their infancy;
4. inordinate health care costs hobble the economy's international competitiveness; and
5. existing arrangements for long-term care are excessively costly and inadequate.

No Consensus on What Should Be Done

Though there is wide agreement on the analysis of the defects in the U.S. health care system, no consensus has as yet developed on what can or should be done to correct these perceived problems. Nevertheless, there is a widely shared belief that fundamental reform is needed. A *Wall Street Journal*/NBC News poll of registered voters in June 1991 found that, given a list of six pressing issues, 4 voters in 10 selected health care (along with the economy) far more than issues such as education, drugs and crime, homelessness, and the environment. Large majorities of both Democrats and Republicans favored strong government action — either by requiring employers to provide health care for their employees or through a government program.

The goal is to develop a health care system that makes quality, affordable care available to all Americans. A number of proposals have been presented for achieving this goal, and others can be anticipated in the coming months.

There is some evidence that one approach is beginning to be favored by many, but not all, of those actively promoting health care reform. Often referred to as "play or pay," this approach is based on the requirement that employers either provide health care benefits for their employees or pay into a public fund that will do so.

It is not possible at this stage to predict the exact contours of the proposals that will be put forth. It is possible, however, to suggest the goals that these proposals must achieve if they are to deal with the major defects in the current U.S. health care system. The members of the Committee on New American Realities — leaders of business, labor, agriculture, and academic institutions — endorse the following goals as essential elements of national health care reform.

Universal coverage. If the program does not achieve universal coverage all at once, it should have a specific timetable for doing so within a few years. The uninsured can be divided into two main categories — the employed and the nonemployed. The program should include specific measures for covering both groups.

A basic level of comprehensive benefits. For benefits to be comprehensive, they should include, at the very least, preventive care, necessary medical care in all appropriate settings, hospitalization, and long-term care in the patient's home and in a nursing home.

Built-in cost controls. High on the list of such controls is a national cap on health care expenditures that, it is anticipated, would provide the ultimate discipline for avoiding excessive health care spending. Subsidiary to this global spending limitation would be fee schedules, a system for determining hospital reimbursement, encouragement of managed care, medical technology assessment, controls on capital expenditures, negotiation of uniform payments to providers, and specific ways of minimizing administrative costs.

Improvements in the quality of care. A specific focus on quality is essential to assure that people get the right treatment. To make certain that there is more than just lip-service to this goal, it is essential that an administrative unit or a commission — or preferably both — be established and charged with the responsibility of enhancing quality in every aspect of health care.

Long-term care. An important component of national health care reform, long-term care should be available to people of all ages who meet the requirements for functional impairment. It should include community-based home and nursing home care. To reduce the cost and improve the quality of long-term care, case management should be an important feature of the program. The program should be financed by a combination of public and private financing.

Affordable, adequate and equitable financing. In global terms, "affordable" can be viewed as the amount the nation thinks it can spend on health care. Affordable can also be considered only as it relates to public expenditures for health care. Finally, it is important to take into account whether the various participants and payers will consider that they can afford the financial obligations they will be required to undertake.

The amount of funds that can be judged "adequate" must be sufficient to pay for the benefits to which the program entitles participants. The costs should be estimated realistically in light of the nature and scope of the benefits offered, the necessity to assure quality care and reasonable payments for the services of providers.

It will not be easy to obtain agreement on what constitutes "equitable" financing. One principle that has had considerable support in the past is that individual payment requirements should be based on ability to pay. Any cost sharing should not be so costly in relation to income or health care condition that it prevents some people from getting needed care.

A favorable impact on the competitiveness of the American economy. A requirement that all employers carry a fair share of health care costs will eliminate the unfair advantage that employers who do not pay for their employees' health care now have over competitors who carry such costs. If the program includes a strong element of cost control, this will enhance American industry's competitiveness in international markets.

Compatibility with American traditions, principles and institutions. For far-reaching health care reform to be adopted and then made effective, it will have to have broad public understanding and support. It will require federal legislation that will have to pass both Houses of Congress and be signed by the President. This will not happen unless there is a broad consensus that the reform is necessary and will be viable. Elements such as a public-private program, opportunity for choice and emphasis on quality, affordability and equity are in the American tradition and are compatible with cherished American principles.

The nation has an opportunity — perhaps unprecedented — to reform the health care system in ways that will greatly enhance its effectiveness and equity and ensure access to health care that many Americans lack today. Organizations like the National Planning Association can make a significant contribution by informing people about the problems we face in health care and the ways in which we can meet them. If there is both broad public understanding of the issues and a political will for action, we can achieve a system that assures affordable quality health care to all Americans.

Note

There are differing views among the members of the Committee on New American Realities concerning specific proposals for reform of the U.S. health care system. Some NAR Committee members do not agree with all of the recommendations presented in this report. Nevertheless, they do agree to its issuance in the hope that it will contribute to public discussion of these key issues.

About the Author

Bert Seidman is a consultant to the National Council of Senior Citizens. He also serves as a board member of the National Council on the Aging, a vice president of the National Consumer League and advisory director of the International Foundation of Employee Benefit Plans. Retiring after 42 years with the AFL-CIO as Director of Occupational Safety, Health and Social Security, Mr. Seidman had policy responsibilities in fields such as health care, social security, pensions, and unemployment insurance. He has served on a number of advisory bodies, including the Task Force on Medicaid and Related Programs, the Advisory Council on Social Security, the Health Insurance Benefits Advisory Council (formally an advisory body on Medicare and Medicaid) and the Prospective Payment Assessment Commission (current advisory group on hospital care under Medicare), the Brookings Institution Advisory Panel on Long-Term Care, and the National Advisory Committee to the Robert Wood Johnson Foundation on Community Programs for Affordable Health Care. Mr. Seidman is a member of the National Managed Health Care Council and the Wellness Council of America.

Any opinions expressed are those of the author and are not necessarily endorsed by the National Council of Senior Citizens or any other organization with which Mr. Seidman has a current or past association.

Acknowledgments

The National Planning Association wishes to express its appreciation for the generous financial support of GTE in making possible the publication of *Curing U.S. Health Care Ills*. It is through such support that NPA is able to advance public discussion and aid public-private policy formulation on vital issues like health care reform.

Chapter I

Introduction

America's health care system is in deep trouble. Most Americans are dissatisfied with it and want a fundamental change. What should be done and how changes should be carried out, however, are complex issues not easily resolved.

The dissatisfaction of nearly all Americans with their health care system stems from its impingement on all sectors of American society. Such overwhelming discontent is not surprising since the United States has the most expensive health care system in the industrialized world (Chart 1.1), and these spiraling costs are jeopardizing the coverage of the majority of Americans. Yet, except for South Africa, the United States is the only

Chart 1.1: Comparison of Health Care Expenditures, Selected OECD Countries, 1987
(As Percentage of Gross Domestic Product)

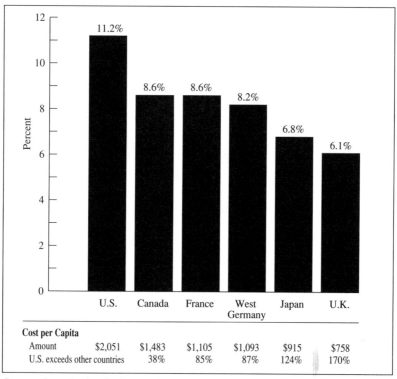

Source: Organization for Economic Cooperation and Development, 1989.

industrialized country with a significant proportion of its population lacking health care coverage. The demand for health care reform is widespread and insistent. Poll after poll has demonstrated that the American people want fundamental reform of the health care system and that they are ready for major change. According to a recent poll, 89 percent of Americans believe the current health care system needs to be radically altered. This is indeed the time for action.

Perceptions about Health Care

Employers have seen expenditures for health care for their employees and families rise unrelentingly over a long period of time. Moreover, the efforts of many firms to restrain health care costs have had little or no effect. Year after year, employers have faced double-digit health care cost inflation — and there is no letup in sight. Year after year, the increase in medical costs has greatly exceeded the increase in the Consumer Price Index (CPI) (Chart 1.2, page 4). These ever mounting costs have weakened U.S. competitiveness in markets both at home and abroad.

Leaders of American labor have concluded that the employment-based health care system in the United States that provides health care coverage for most American workers may be collapsing. Many workers, union and nonunion, have seen long-established health care coverage sharply reduced. Some unions have reluctantly decided to sacrifice wages or other benefits to maintain hard-won health care benefits.

The federal government has sought to introduce cost controls in its programs, especially Medicare which provides health care for the elderly and the severely disabled. Cost restraints have had some impact on Medicare hospital inpatient care. Medicare outpatient cost controls are soon to take effect, and there is good reason to think they will have some beneficial impact. Despite such efforts, however, federal health care costs continue to rise rapidly.

One state after another has faced fiscal crises, especially in the past few years, to which rapidly escalating health care costs have largely contributed. For most states, the Medicaid costs that they share with the federal government have become one of their largest spending categories. They have found that, to meet their Medicaid obligations while maintaining a balance in their overall budgets, they have had to reduce their spending for non-health programs.

3

Chart 1.2: Consumer Price Index Increases versus Medical Costs

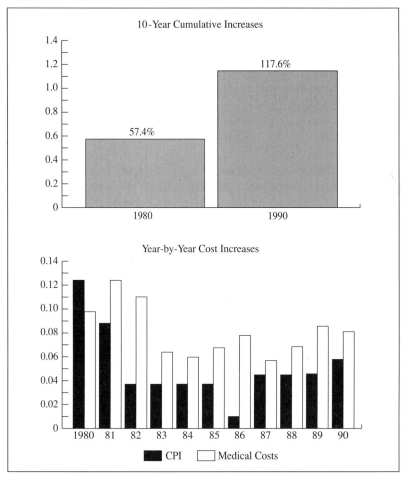

Source: U.S. Bureau of Labor Statistics.

There was a time when the lack of health care coverage for some Americans was either largely unknown or ignored. This is no longer true. The fact that a significant proportion of Americans do not have access to health care is widely publicized and the subject of much public discussion.

Estimates vary as to how many Americans lack health care coverage, but there are at least 31 million, approximately one-sixth of the population under 65 years of age. Some estimates are as high as 40 million.

In addition, according to 1990 data from the Census Bureau, about 42 million lacked coverage for at least 7 months during a 28-month period. Tens of millions have inadequate coverage, the exact number depending on how "inadequate" is defined. It has become increasingly evident that the technological medical marvels now common in U.S. hospitals permit people to be kept alive at enormous expense and often in great pain and discomfort when they would prefer to be permitted to die in peace with as little pain and as much comfort as possible. The growing interest in living wills and proposals for state legislation to deal with artificial prolongation of life attest to the concern that it is not only unnecessarily costly but also ethically wrong and often cruel to prolong life artificially.

Despite the significant extent of noncoverage, most Americans have some kind of coverage for acute medical care, through their employment for those under 65 years and through Medicare for the elderly. But very few Americans have any coverage for chronic or long-term health care — either home or nursing home care. Yet, with the aging population, the need for long-term care is rapidly expanding. Our largest long-term care program is Medicaid, a welfare program that requires middle-income patients to become paupers to obtain its assistance.

A Consensus about What Is Wrong with U.S. Health Care

Until recent years, observers of the health care scene had conflicting ideas about the U.S. health care system. Some maintained that it was "the best health care system in the world" and needed little, if any, change. Others were much more critical. They felt that certain features, especially the predominant fee-for-service method of paying doctors and reimbursement of all hospital spending without restriction, made the system far too costly. Critics described the prevailing organization and delivery of care as ineffective and favored alternative systems such as prepaid group practice plans (now called health maintenance organizations or HMOs). They also criticized the system because of its failure to provide adequately for some Americans, especially the poor and minorities.

However, in recent years, a remarkable consensus has developed about what is wrong with the nation's health care system. The main conclusions are that:

1. health care costs are excessive and for many years have been rising far faster than the overall inflation rate;

2. depending on estimation methods, 31 million to 40 million people have no health care coverage and at least as many have inadequate coverage;
3. in important respects, quality of care is unsatisfactory and measures to assess it, the only basis on which improvements can be effected, are in their infancy;
4. inordinate health care costs hobble the economy's international competitiveness; and
5. existing arrangements for long-term care are excessively costly and inadequate.

No Consensus on What Should Be Done

Though there is wide agreement on the analysis of the defects in the U.S. health care system, no consensus has as yet developed on what can or should be done to correct these perceived problems. Nevertheless, there is a widely shared belief that fundamental reform is needed. A *Wall Street Journal*/NBC News poll of registered voters in June 1991 found that, given a list of six pressing issues, 4 voters in 10 selected health care (along with the economy) far more than issues such as education, drugs and crime, homelessness, and the environment. Large majorities of both Democrats and Republicans favored strong government action — either by requiring employers to provide health care for their employees or through a government program.

A number of groups have developed proposals, some of which are far-reaching while others involve much less change from the existing system. Some of the proposals have been set out in considerable detail, while others are, at this time, stated only in very general terms. However, some patterns can be discerned from these proposals, and they are discussed later.

Chapter II

Costs and Expenditures

Of even more direct concern to most Americans than the lack of access to health care for some is that runaway health care inflation is jeopardizing the health care coverage of the majority of Americans. The rapid rise in health care costs is the most important single factor engendering dissatisfaction with the current system.

Distribution of Health Care Expenditures

Spending on health care has risen faster than the gross national product in all but three years since 1960. In 1989, national health care expenditures rose to $604.1 billion, 11.1 percent more than the previous year. Following a two-decade upward trend, health care spending reached 11.6 percent of GNP compared with 11.2 percent in 1988 and only 5.3 percent in 1960. U.S. health care costs are still rising rapidly and far outpacing GNP. According to the Office of National Health Statistics, health spending in 1990 was $671.0 billion, 12.2 percent of GNP — an increase of three times the average of the past 30 years. The U.S. percentage is significantly higher than that of any other country in the world, almost 50 percent more than that of members of the Organization for Economic Cooperation and Development (OECD) (see Chart 1.1, page 2).

More than two-fifths of U.S. health care expenditures are paid by individuals, and this share has increased since 1980. The rest is divided almost evenly between business and government. Between 1980 and 1987, the share of individuals increased from 38.4 to 41.5 percent, government's share dropped from 32.1 to 29.9 percent, and the share of business fell from 28.8 to 27.9 percent.

In addition to these direct sources of financing, there are important indirect sources. In 1988, hospitals provided $8.3 billion of care for uninsured patients that was reflected in the charges to other payers. Another indirect source of health care spending takes the form of business tax deductions for contributions to employment-based health plans, which amounted to $33 billion in 1990.

There has been a marked change in recent years in the distribution of hospital and nonhospital expenditures. Hospital expenditures in each year between 1982 and 1988 were 4.3 percent (or slightly less) of GNP. The entire increase in the proportion of health care expenditures to GNP was attributable to nonhospital expenditures, which steadily rose from 5.9 percent of GNP in 1982 to 6.7 percent in 1988. This undoubtedly reflected the fact that the focus of health care cost-restraint efforts in both the public and private sectors was primarily on hospital inpatient costs.

8

Health Care Inflation

From 1973 to 1988, national health expenditures grew by 429 percent, more than two and one-half times the general inflation rate as measured by the CPI. Employer health care costs increased even more — by 602 percent over the same period.

Throughout the 1980s, both unions and employers made determined efforts to hold down health care costs. But it was a losing battle. A survey by the Wyatt Company of more than 900 employer-sponsored medical plans showed an average increase of 21 percent in annual costs of medical benefits from 1987 to 1989. Health care costs for employers from 1985 to 1989 were two to four times the overall inflation rate shown by the CPI (Chart 2.1). This was all the more shocking because of the significant shift in costs to employees during that period (see Chart 2.2, page 13).

Chart 2.1: Employer Costs for Health Care Compared to the CPI, 1985-89

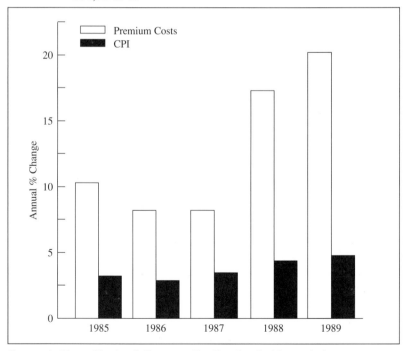

Source: A. Foster Higgins & Company, Inc. Reprinted with permission.

Health care spending has been consuming a constantly increasing share of corporate operating profits. In 1965, spending for health care services was under 10 percent of corporate operating profits. In 1988, it was estimated to be nearly 50 percent, and it may be even higher today. Half of the uninsured are employed by small firms. The small business enterprises that do provide health care coverage have been particularly hard hit by runaway health care inflation. Small businesses generally have to pay higher insurance rates than large firms and are less likely to be able to institute cost control measures. The result is that their premiums average 40 percent more per person covered and have been increasing faster than premiums in large businesses. These increases make it very difficult for small firms that provide health care benefits to maintain them. Further, knowledge of this experience makes other small firms not offering health care coverage very reluctant to do so.

Measured by both per capita spending and proportion of GNP, the United States spends far more for health care than any other industrialized country. In 1987, the United States spent 11.2 percent of its gross domestic product for health care. As Chart 1.1, page 2, shows, Canada and France each spent 8.6 percent; West Germany, 8.2 percent; Japan, 6.8 percent; and the United Kingdom, 6.1 percent. Indeed, in some countries, including Sweden and Germany, the proportion of GNP spent on health care has actually dropped. Even more significant perhaps was the percentage by which the U.S. per capita cost for health care ($2,051 in 1987) exceeded the per capita costs for the other countries, ranging from 38 percent for Canada — which has the second most expensive health care system in the world — to 170 percent for the United Kingdom.

Health care administrative costs in the United States are almost nine times higher than in Canada. In 1989, the expense-to-premium ratio of commercial insurers in the United States was just under 27 percent compared with only 3 percent in Canada. One reason for this difference is the existence in the United States of over 1,200 private insurance companies with many duplications of sales staffs, billing, premium payments, vendor payments, and reimbursements to consumers, which add tremendously to the administrative costs of the U.S. health care system.

Canada's provincial governments pay all major health care expenses for Canadians; thus they have no marketing expenses. Every Canadian is entitled by law to the statutory health care benefits, which are the same for everyone. This eliminates the need to determine eligibility or coverage. Because any differences in premiums or taxes paid are related only to family size and not to risk status, the costs of estimating risk status are removed. Further, claims payment is much simpler and therefore less costly under the Canadian system. Hospitals, physicians and other providers are relieved of complying with the requirements of a myriad of insurers as well as of the billing of their patients. This huge disparity in administrative costs between the United States and Canada means that in Canada almost all health care dollars are spent for treatment of sick patients, while in the United States more than one in four health care dollars is wasted on administrative expenses and marketing.

A study from the *New England Journal of Medicine* reported that in 1985, per capita expenditure for physicians' services was $347 in the United States and $202 (U.S. dollars) in Canada, even though the U.S. per capita quantity of physicians' services was somewhat less than three-fourths the Canadian level. Higher expenditures on physicians' services in the United States were entirely attributable to the fact that physicians' fees were more than twice as high in this country than in Canada. Yet, U.S. physicians' net income was only about one-third higher. The main reason for the disparity between U.S. and Canadian spending for physicians' care was that U.S. physicians use nearly twice as many resources to produce a given quantity of services.

A recent joint Canadian-U.S. study shows that although on a per capita basis the United States spent close to 50 percent more on hospitals than Canada in 1985, public and private hospital care cost controls in the United States have not been as effective as government controls in Canada (Newhouse et al., 1988). These are exercised by provincial ministries of health, which approve and fund hospital operating budgets that are annually negotiated between the ministry and the hospital. The ministry's approval is also required for new facilities and equipment and major renovations. Another reason for higher hospital costs in the United States is the widespread proliferation of high technology inpatient care that has not been duplicated in Canada. The impact of this development on the quality of care is debatable, but it has certainly contributed to the high cost of hospital care in the United States.

Cost Shifting

In an effort to escape ever mounting health care costs, there has been a tremendous amount of cost shifting. As Professor Uwe Reinhardt of

Princeton University observed in a recent speech, "the system passes around patients and costs like so many hot potatoes."

From government to private payers. Hospitals and other providers do not charge all payers the same amount. A 1982 study by the Urban Institute of 128 private nonprofit hospitals found that:

- commercial insurer payments were 26.7 percent higher than the average cost;
- Medicare payments were about equal to the average cost; and
- Medicaid payments were 10 percent lower than the average cost.

In 1982, Medicare, which used to pay hospitals on a cost basis, shifted to a system that pays all hospitals at a pre-established rate. The same system has been adopted in a number of states for Medicaid payments to hospitals. While Medicare and Medicaid spending has continued to rise, Medicare's system of cost restraint has kept its payments to hospitals from rising as fast as the payments of other payers. Because the hospitals contend that Medicare prepayment rates are not sufficient, whenever possible they have tried to get other payers to make up the difference. In addition, Medicare pays only for services rendered to beneficiaries, which excludes uncompensated care for the uninsured. These costs are then shifted to other payers. Further, hospitals claim that Medicaid payments do not cover the full cost of Medicaid patients and that Medicaid payments have declined in relation to cost. This has also resulted in cost shifting to other payers.

From the federal government to state and local government. During the 1980s, large numbers of people removed from Medicaid eligibility sought medical care from public hospitals mainly funded by state and local governments. Many of these hospitals have been under severe fiscal pressure and have had to close whole wings or departments including, in some instances, emergency services. The Medicare prepayment system has resulted in reduced length of stay and earlier discharges for Medicare patients. For some Medicare beneficiaries, post-discharge care has involved services paid wholly or partially from state or local funds.

From employers to employees. Employers, faced with rapidly expanding health care costs, have been shifting part of those costs to their employees. According to the Employee Benefit Research Institute, even though employer contributions to employer-sponsored health insurance plans rose very rapidly from 1982 to 1988, employee contributions grew four times as fast. Employers have shifted costs to employees by requiring employees to pay part of the premium cost or by raising deductibles and co-payments, by curtailing covered services, by eliminating or restricting family coverage, by reducing or eliminating retiree coverage, and by tightening length of service requirements (Chart 2.2). As a result of such impediments to health coverage, the Service Employees International Union found in a 1989 survey of its members that middle income workers were at risk for medical payments as high as one-fifth of after-tax income and low income workers over one-third.

From large to small employers and vice versa. To the extent that large employers are able to reduce their costs by obtaining discounted rates from health care providers or insurers, smaller firms that provide health care benefits for their employees are unable to get such discounts and thus face higher premiums. Some small firms, faced with demands for sharp increases in premiums that they regard as unaffordable, have either drastically curtailed their health care benefits or dropped them altogether.

Chart 2.2: Changes in Health Insurance Cost Sharing Since 1987

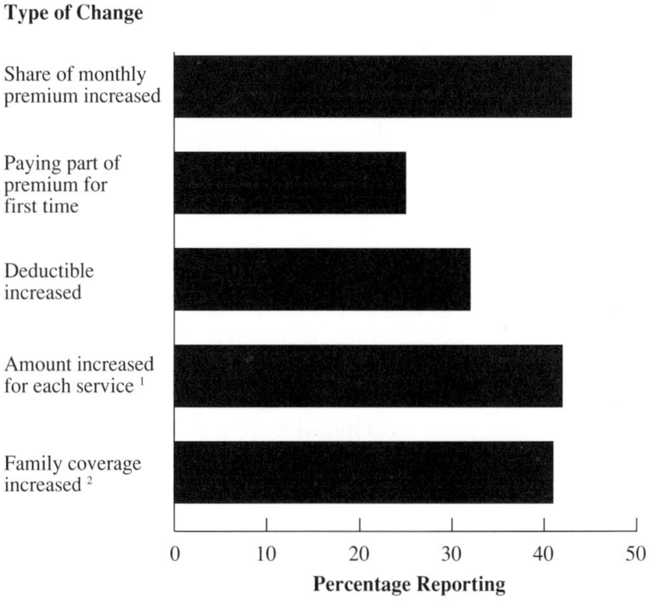

Type of Change

- Share of monthly premium increased
- Paying part of premium for first time
- Deductible increased
- Amount increased for each service [1]
- Family coverage increased [2]

Percentage Reporting (0, 10, 20, 30, 40, 50)

[1] Service refers to each time the respondent receives health care covered by insurance, such as a visit to the doctor.

[2] Family coverage is considered to be provided under respondent's insurance plan.

Source: Employee Benefit Research Institute, *Public Attitudes on Health Insurance Provision* (Washington, D.C.: EBRI/The Gallup Organization, Inc., August 1989).

However, many small (and some large) employers have never provided health care coverage for their employees. The health care costs of these employees, to the extent that they cannot meet them out-of-pocket, are absorbed by health care providers. The costs of employees of firms that do not provide coverage are ultimately reflected in the rates and premiums paid by the employers whose employees are covered.

Shift to Self-Insurance

In recent years, many employers, especially large firms, have sought to reduce their health care costs by switching from contracting with insurance companies or Blue Cross-Blue Shield to insure risk to contracting with them to administer programs that the employers self-insure.

This has a number of cost advantages for employers. Self-insurance relieves the employer from paying the insurer's premium, which includes the amount the insurer retains (the retention rate) over and above the cost. In addition, federal law exempts self-insured firms from requirements under state law to provide certain types of benefits — such as chiropractic care, substance abuse treatment and a number of other specific health care benefits — that states have mandated health insurance companies to provide in all their employment-based plans.

Retiree Health Care

Retiree health care costs are affected by all the factors that influence the health care costs of active workers plus others relating especially to retirees. These include the aging of the population (greater longevity that adds to the length of the period in retirement), the need of older persons for more medical care, and the continued trend toward early retirement. According to the General Accounting Office, employers paid $9 billion in 1988 for retiree health benefits and are projected to pay $22 billion by 2005.

Under a new financial rule announced by the Financial Accounting Standards Board (the private group under the aegis of the Securities and Exchange Commission that makes financial rules for companies), beginning in 1993 companies will have to deduct from current earnings part of the cost of health care benefits that they anticipate paying for future retirees. This is contrary to the current accounting practices of almost all companies. The overwhelming majority of firms have been accounting for retiree health care costs on a pay-as-you-go basis. No one knows the extent

14

of liability under the new FASB rule, but it has been estimated from over $200 billion to as high as $2 trillion. Hardest hit will be companies with many retirees and an aging workforce. A survey of large employers by Towers, Perrin, Foster & Crosby, a benefit consulting firm, found that if the rule had been in effect in 1990, the amount that the average surveyed company would have had to set aside per employee would have jumped from $340 to $2,500.

Employers can be expected to exert tremendous pressure to reduce their liabilities by cutting back on or eliminating future retiree health care benefits, while unions will do everything possible to maintain them. According to a survey by Buck Consultants, 82 percent of 236 companies surveyed reserve the right to change or terminate retiree coverage. The question of whether employers have the right to withdraw promised health care benefits for current retirees and, if so, under what circumstances is in litigation. Whatever the outcome, it would not appear to affect the right of employers to reduce benefits for future retirees and their dependents. Therefore, health care benefits for retirees will continue to be a contentious issue between labor and management, especially in the wake of the new FASB rule.

Reasons for Excessive Health Care Costs

Unlike many other countries, the United States does not fix overall limits on health care spending. Decisions as to what care will be provided and how much will be paid are dispersed among countless numbers of providers, payers, insurers, and consumers. Some may have reasons for restraining costs, but others may be motivated to expand them, and no one has enough influence to establish a limitation on total health care spending.

Another reason for high health care costs in the United States is that, with limited exceptions, providers determine both the demand levels and the payment levels for medical care. Physicians play an especially crucial role in this aspect of health care. Except for the initial contact that patients make with the health care system, physicians largely determine utilization of medical care. They determine both outpatient and inpatient treatment, tests given, surgery performed, drugs prescribed, post-hospital treatment, and practically all other aspects of health care utilization. The role doctors play in determining the demand and thus the cost of medical care is all the more crucial because there has been an increasing trend for doctors to practice in narrow specialties and sub-specialties that involve highly costly procedures and technology rather than in preventive and primary care.

15

In most cases, providers have determined how much they were paid. Doctors set their fee levels and hospitals set their rates with very few constraints. However, exceptions to this pattern are beginning to emerge. Payment systems have been set up affecting both hospitals and physicians under Medicare. Physicians' payments are predetermined in HMOs and preferred provider organizations (PPOs). Some states have enacted rate-setting for hospital care. Despite these developments, however, most providers still have no restrictions on what they can charge for their services.

The lack of an integrated health care system (except for public programs) results in very high administrative costs. The great disparity in administrative costs between Canada and the United States has already been discussed. There is a similar difference between administrative costs of private insurers and those under Medicare. In 1989, the expense-to-premium ratio for Medicare was only 2.3 percent compared with 26.9 percent for private insurers. What distinguishes both Medicare and Canada's health care system from medical care under commercial insurance is that the public systems involve a single payer and no marketing costs, which greatly reduce costs that are unrelated to the delivery of health care.

Currently there are no controls on capital costs for health care facilities and equipment. It is estimated that an average of one-third of all hospital beds remain unoccupied each day. The American Hospital Association reported in *National Hospital Panel Survey* that in 1989 hospital payments and depreciation costs for capital projects, reflecting spending for buildings and equipment in prior years, amounted to $16.6 billion, up from $4.9 billion in 1980 and $11.1 billion in 1985. In the case of private payers, these costs are simply reflected in hospital rates. Medicare divides its payments between operating and investment costs. Although there are controls on operating costs, Medicare pays hospitals 85 percent of actual capital costs based on the proportion of Medicare patients to total patients. There is widespread concern that the present system of paying for hospitals' capital spending is wasteful because all capital spending, whether duplicative or not and whether needed or not, is reimbursed by public and private payers. Another important factor encouraging the overuse of expensive medical technology is a reimbursement system that has always paid more to doctors performing sophisticated procedures involving costly medical equipment than to doctors who provide more routine medical care.

There is a growing consensus that a significant proportion of medical care is inappropriate, excessive and even harmful. This affects both the quality and the cost of medical care.

A Rand Corporation study lists a significant number of questionable and unjustified medical procedures, including:

- 14 percent of all coronary bypass operations at an average cost of $37,000;
- 32 percent of arterial balloon operations at an average cost of $9,000; and
- 17 percent of upper gastrointestinal examinations.

Much unnecessary care results from the practice of so-called defensive medicine by physicians who fear malpractice litigation. Doctors order costly, unnecessary tests and treatment to cover themselves in the event that they have to defend themselves in a malpractice suit brought by a patient. Malpractice insurance rates in the United States are by far the highest in the world. The trend of malpractice costs has been sharply upward since at least the 1970s. One of the periods of sharpest escalation was during the mid-1970s when, responding to concern about the unavailability and increasing cost of medical malpractice insurance, 49 states enacted various reforms. In 1986, the General Accounting Office issued a report on the experience of six states (Arkansas, California, Florida, Indiana, New York, and North Carolina) that had instituted tort reforms aimed at assuring availability and reducing the cost of malpractice insurance. The GAO found that malpractice insurance rates increased sharply from 1980 to 1986. The GAO also reported that an earlier study (1982) found no significant effects of the reforms on frequency of claims or amount of awards. While more far-reaching reforms have been suggested, including no-fault, arbitration and social insurance proposals, no consensus has as yet developed on dealing with this problem.

Providers, especially physicians, have found a number of ways to "game the system," and this has resulted in higher costs for purchasers of care. Such practices of physicians and the terms that are used to designate them include:

- unbundling — coding a surgical operation (e.g., a hysterectomy) as a number of separate procedures;
- exploding — itemizing a series of tests that are done on a single sample of blood; and
- upcoding — for example, coding the removal of a three millimeter mole as a two centimeter mole.

Most hospital patients receive extremely technical and detailed billing statements that the average person finds almost impossible to understand, much less to check for accuracy. Yet, for those insurers and payers who have checked such bills, errors have been found that almost always have resulted in higher payments.

Another factor adding to costs is that hospitals in many communities compete not on the basis of price but on the basis of which hospital can provide the most sophisticated services and the latest technologically advanced equipment. The United States has a well developed system for testing the efficiency and therapeutic value of drugs but no comparable approach for assessing new medical technology, although such proposals have been offered for two or more decades. The problem is made worse because no measures are taken to assure that expensive medical technology is fully utilized. Often the same equipment is used at far less than capacity in facilities that are close enough to each other to warrant sharing of the equipment at much reduced cost. It has been found that infrequent use of highly technological medical procedures not only inflates the cost of the treatment but also detracts from its quality and may even threaten the safety of patients.

Impact on Competitiveness of the U.S. Economy

A major result of health care inflation is its harmful impact on U.S. competitiveness. American employers are increasingly concerned that the heavy and ever mounting costs of the U.S. health care system that they bear — costs that they share more and more with their employees — put them in a highly disadvantageous position vis-a-vis their foreign competitors in countries with national health care systems. The additional health care costs borne by American industry can be attributed to a number of factors. Among the most important are the following.

Inflation. Year after year, U.S. health care costs have not just been higher than those of other industrialized countries, but they have also been rising more rapidly. Thus, the disadvantage of American firms has been growing (Chart 2.3).

Unnecessary care. In recent years, there has been voluminous documentation of the high number of unnecessary tests, treatment and surgery that is endemic in the U.S. health care system. In part, these needless procedures result from the way we still pay for most hospital and doctor services — the more services provided, the higher the payment. In part, the procedures result from the practice of defensive medicine by doctors fearful of malpractice litigation. The net effect is to add greatly to total health care spending in the United States.

Administrative costs. As already mentioned, the U.S. health care system involving hundreds of insurers, each with different forms and bureaucratic requirements and the need to check on eligibility and coverage for each health care encounter for each patient, creates inordinate administrative costs that never arise in other countries. In addition, the competition of insurers and providers for the health care dollar involves large marketing costs that are also not present in other countries.

Cost shifting. Still another major factor is the shifting to private payers of the costs of care for uninsured patients, however inadequate that care may be. Because countries with universal entitlement to health care have virtually no uninsured citizens, there is no such cost shifting to the foreign competitors of U.S. firms.

In 1988, Chrysler estimated its health care costs at $700 per vehicle (Chart 2.4, page 20). Comparable costs in other industrialized countries were: France, $375; Germany, $337; Japan, $246; and Canada, $223.

Walter F. Williams, chairman and chief executive officer of the Bethlehem Steel Corporation, recently stated that health care costs in the

Chart 2.3: Total Health Care Expenditures, Selected OECD Countries, 1970-89
(As Percentage of GDP)

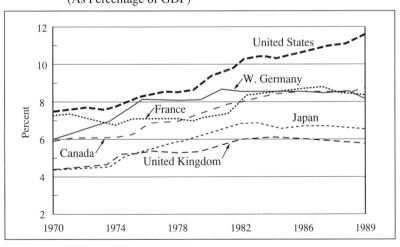

Source: *Health OECD, Facts and Trends* (Paris: OECD, forthcoming).

19

Chart 2.4: Health Care Costs per Vehicle, 1988

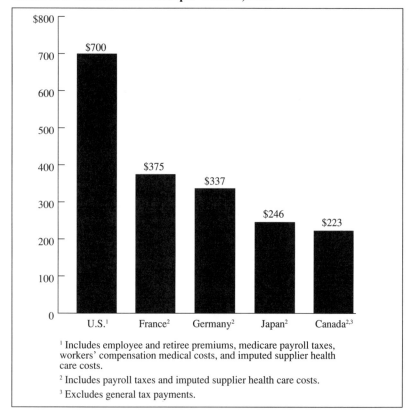

¹ Includes employee and retiree premiums, medicare payroll taxes, workers' compensation medical costs, and imputed supplier health care costs.
² Includes payroll taxes and imputed supplier health care costs.
³ Excludes general tax payments.

Source: Information received from the Chrysler Corporation.

American steel industry have doubled in the past 10 years, reaching 15 percent of total employment costs in 1991. He said that these costs are two to three times as high as those in steel companies abroad and seriously threaten the competitiveness of America's steel industry.

Efforts to Control Health Care Costs

Employers, unions, businesses, and governments, both separately and sometimes in joint efforts, have sought to restrain health care costs. These efforts have been ongoing for a long period of time, but they increased dramatically during the 1980s.

Inpatient hospital care. In that decade for the most part, efforts focused on reducing unnecessary hospitalization and surgery and on controlling hospital costs for inpatient care. It seemed sensible to concentrate on inpatient hospital costs because hospitalization and surgery were the most expensive kinds of care, and it was thought that restraining these costs would have the biggest payoff. A number of measures aimed at reducing hospital costs became quite common in employment-based plans and were generally supported by both management and labor (Chart 2.5). These measures included:

Chart 2.5: Adoption of Cost Management Techniques, 1984-88

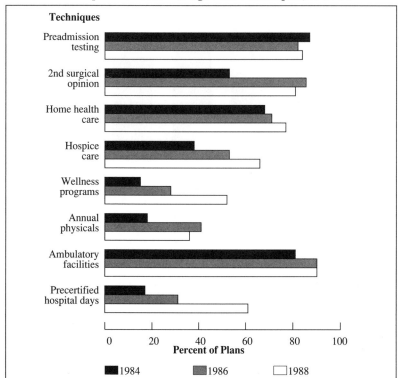

Source: Data first published in a 1988 survey by the Wyatt Company. Reproduced with permission from EMPLOYEE BENEFITS MANAGEMENT, *Cost Containment, The Health Benefits Challenge of the '90s*, published and copyrighted by the Commerce Clearing House, Inc. (4025 W. Peterson Ave., Chicago, Illinois 60646), January 1990, p. 7.

21

• second opinions for nonemergency surgery;
• preadmission testing;
• preadmission certification (requirement for doctors and hospitals to get insurer approval before a covered patient could be admitted to a hospital);
• monitoring length of stay;
• monitoring hospital billing;
• outpatient surgery; and
• disclosure by insurers and providers of essential data to payers (including both management and labor).

Employers, labor and the two groups in cooperative labor-management programs have had some success in using these measures to hold down health care inflation. In the early 1980s, increases slowed to a more moderate pace (10-12 percent annually), but sharp escalation (in the range of 25-30 percent or more) resumed in 1987, especially in mainly uncontrolled outpatient costs. A survey by A. Foster Higgins & Company of large and medium sized corporations found that health care costs of surveyed corporations rose 17.1 percent in 1990 and nearly doubled from 1985 to 1989 (Chart 2.1, page 9). If dental, vision and hearing coverage are excluded and only traditional medical coverage is considered, the increase was 21.6 percent in 1990. The sharp escalation in costs apparently occurred in outpatient care, which continues to be largely uncontrolled.

Total admissions to community hospitals decreased gradually from about 9.5 million quarterly in 1984 to slightly over 8 million quarterly, or more than 15 percent, by 1990. The length of stay of hospital patients generally declined from 1976 to 1985 and then leveled off between 1985 and 1990. During the latter period, outpatient visits to community hospitals increased from somewhat under 60 million quarterly to over 80 million quarterly, or about 33 percent. The disparity in trends between inpatient and outpatient revenue is even more marked. From 1980 to 1989, hospital inpatient revenue increased from $69 billion to $152 billion, or about 120 percent, while outpatient revenues rose from $10 billion to $43 billion, or 330 percent. Visits to physicians' offices per week declined from 1976 to 1984 but increased somewhat thereafter. Thus, there has been a decided shift since the mid-1980s from inpatient hospitalization to outpatient care both in the hospital and, to a somewhat lesser extent, in the physician's office. It is especially significant that cost control efforts have been largely concentrated on inpatient hospital care with little or no restraint on hospital outpatient costs or physician fees (*Digest of National Health Care Use*, 1990).

Managed care. In the face of constantly escalating costs and the ineffectiveness of earlier health care cost containment measures that focused on reducing hospital spending, employers and unions have turned to "managed care." There is no single accepted definition of managed care. It generally involves deliberate action taken to influence the cost, quality, mode, or site of delivery of health care. As defined in a February 1990 paper of the Health Insurance Association of America (HIAA):

> Managed care systems integrate both the financing and delivery of appropriate health care services to covered individuals by means of the following basic elements: arrangements with selected providers to furnish a comprehensive set of health care services to members; explicit standards for the selection of health care providers; formal programs for ongoing quality assurance and utilization review; and significant financial incentives for members to use the providers and procedures associated with the plan.

Managed care systems take many forms; some are more comprehensive and involve a greater degree of control of utilization and costs than others. Almost 35 million Americans are in health maintenance organizations that provide comprehensive health care for a set fee. Generally, members get all their care from the HMO. A somewhat less organized system is the preferred provider organizations, which cover an even greater number of individuals than HMOs. PPOs generally contract for discounts in return for financial incentives to those they cover to use PPO-designated providers, i.e., hospitals and/or physicians. However, PPO members are not required to get all their care from PPO providers, and many do not. PPOs and other managed care arrangements usually involve discounts, often negotiated by insurers on behalf of purchasers, with networks of providers, hospitals and physicians. Employees are given financial incentives, usually in the form of lower cost-sharing levels, to use the designated providers.

In addition to HMOs and PPOs, some consider any program that includes measures aimed at influencing cost and quality of care as "managed care," while others confine the term to more organized systems of financing and delivery of care. According to the HIAA, in 1982 only 1.5 percent of group health coverage involved a plan with managed care provisions. Just six years later, in 1988, managed care coverage had reached 72 percent.

Wellness and preventive care. The foregoing discussion relates to the treatment of people who are sick. There is increasing recognition that more should be done to forestall illness. Therefore, in recent years, health care programs, including those that are employment-based, have included features such as wellness programs, health promotion, preventive care, and primary care. These are not all the same, and they are somewhat overlapping. Their common goal is to prevent people from getting sick at all or to identify and treat illness in its earliest stage to prevent it from becoming much worse. When these programs are successful, they result not only in healthier people but also in lower medical care costs.

Community coalitions. In some communities, coalitions have been formed to manage health care problems and especially to develop programs aimed at cost restraint. In 1989, there were 129 such coalitions, most of which were organized during the 1980s. In varying configurations, these coalitions include employers (in some cases only employers), providers (hospitals and physicians), unions, and government. Their programs also vary widely. Some are essentially discussion groups; others have tackled specific projects relating to the cost (and less often access and/or quality) of medical care. Most have had little impact on the organization, delivery or cost of medical care in their communities. Their record seems to demonstrate that private groups engaged in voluntary action, even in coalitions of concerned parties, do not wield sufficient power to bring about major health care reform or cost restraint in their communities.

Labor-management cooperation. Increasingly, employers and unions have cooperated in developing specific health care cost restraints to which both parties could agree. Often such labor-management cooperation has begun only after bitter industrial disputes in which health care costs have been a major, or even the single most important, issue. These labor-management programs have been established in a number of industries including auto, communications, steel, men's clothing, and cereal, and some involve state and local public employees and local firms or groups of firms. The labor-management groups have focused on developing programs to control the cost and quality of health care, especially managed care programs that give employees an incentive to use cost-effective providers.

There is a growing consensus, but it is by no means unanimous, that the forces within the private sector are too weak and uncoordinated to control health care costs effectively. Those who have reached this consensus have concluded that health care cost-containment efforts sponsored by a single firm or group of firms, however well intentioned, cannot generate sufficient bargaining power with insurers or providers to restrain health care inflation on a lasting basis. They feel that government action will be required to either replace or supplement private efforts. However, not all share this view. Some in both employer and insurer circles believe that wide application of managed care will be sufficient to hold down health care cost increases to acceptable levels.

State action. In addition to private sector efforts to reduce health care inflation, there has also been government action at both the federal and state levels. The federal government has confined its role to Medicare, the major health care program it administers and finances. Some states have instituted hospital rate-setting programs that apply to all payments, both public and private. Although there are considerable differences in how these programs operate, they are often referred to as "all payer systems" because they apply the hospital payment rate that they have determined to all purchasers of hospital services. In general, these state programs have been unable to stem the tide of health care inflation, but the record has been better in states with rate-setting programs than in those without them.

Chapter III

Access to Care

Most people in the United States receive some kind of health care coverage at their place of work. The exceptions for those with health care coverage are the elderly and severely disabled under Medicare, very low income people under Medicaid and the relatively small number of people who purchase health insurance on an individual basis. But a significant minority of Americans exist without any health care coverage, public or private, and their lack of access to health care has become a matter of growing public concern.

Extent of Noncoverage

The exact number of people in the United States who lack health care coverage is not known. As pointed out earlier, estimates range from 31 million to 40 million or more. Based on the March 1990 Current Population Survey, the Employee Benefit Research Institute reported that in 1989, 34.4 million Americans, nearly 16 percent of the under 65 population, said they had no private health insurance and were ineligible for any public program that financed medical care. The number of uninsured increased by 1.1 million from 1988 to 1989 (EBRI, April 1991).

In addition, in April 1990, the Census Bureau reported that 63 million people (25 percent of the population) lacked insurance protection for substantial periods of time during a recent 28-month period. Of this number, about two-thirds lacked coverage for at least 7 months.

With regard to the one-time estimate of 34.4 million without coverage, more than one-half were workers; adding those who lived in a worker's family brings the proportion of total noncoverage to about 82 percent. Most nonworking uninsured were children (nearly 10 million or 28.7 percent). Less than 17 percent (5.7 million) were nonworking adults (Chart 3.1, page 28).

As expected, the uninsured are more likely to be low income or poor than is the rest of the population. For 1988, 22 percent of the total population, but 46 percent of the uninsured, were in families with less than $5,000 per family member. Thirty percent of the uninsured were poor compared with 13 percent of the total population (EBRI, Sept. 1990).

In the same year, 14 percent of the white population was uninsured compared with 23 percent of blacks and 21 percent of other ethnic groups. A different tabulation for 1988 showed noncoverage was 60 percent higher for Hispanics than for blacks (EBRI, Sept. 1990).

Chart 3.1: Nonelderly Population without Health Insurance, by Own Work Status, 1989

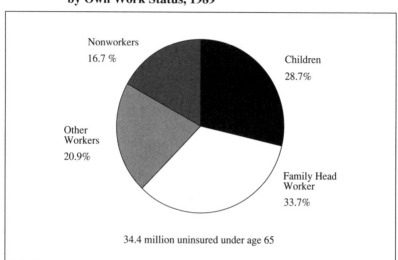

Nonworkers
16.7 %

Children
28.7%

Other
Workers
20.9%

Family Head
Worker
33.7%

34.4 million uninsured under age 65

Source: Employee Benefit Research Institute, *Uninsured in the United States: The Nonelderly Population without Health Insurance - Analysis of the March 1990 Current Population Survey* (Washington, D.C., April 1991).

In 1988, 15 percent of all workers had no health insurance, while 73 percent were covered by their own employer's plan (56 percent) or as a dependent of a covered worker (17 percent). More than three-fourths of uncovered workers were steadily employed throughout the year, and more than one-half were steadily employed in full-time, full-year jobs. Sixty-three percent of uncovered workers earned less than $10,000. Lack of coverage was concentrated in retail trade (23 percent), services (23 percent), manufacturing (13 percent), construction (10 percent), and self-employment (13 percent). Especially high noncoverage was found in agriculture (42 percent) and personal services (32 percent). About one-half of uninsured workers were in firms with fewer than 25 employees (EBRI, Sept. 1990).

In 1988, 15 percent of children under age 15 were uninsured. A different set of Census data compiled by the Population Reference Bureau indicates a somewhat higher noncoverage rate for 18 years of age or younger. From 1986 to 1990, one-fifth of children in that age group lacked coverage (about one-fourth for blacks and one-third for Hispanics), and this number increased slightly in 1990. In poor families, 28 percent of children were not covered, and in near-poor families, 30 percent. The somewhat higher percentage in the near-poor families is attributable to the larger Medicaid coverage among the poor. About one-third of all uninsured children live in poor families. A noteworthy finding is that children in poor families are less likely to be covered if the family head has a job. Nearly one-half of all poor children in families headed by full-time, full-year steadily employed workers were uninsured because they were less likely to qualify for Medicaid than were children in families without full-time workers.

As noted earlier, the extent of inadequate coverage depends on how "inadequate" is defined, but it is generally acknowledged that the number with inadequate coverage is at least equal to the number with no coverage. Perceptions of inadequacy may be even greater than the reality. According to a poll published by the *Los Angeles Times* in 1990, one-half of all Americans believed they could not afford good care if they became critically ill. The same poll found that one in four people put off medical treatment because they could not afford it.

Almost all Americans feel that the nation should be taking steps as quickly as possible to assure universal access to basic health care. But regardless of how widely and sincerely this view is held, the trend is in the other direction. In recent years, noncoverage has been growing, not declining, while health care costs have been rising as a proportion of GNP. According to the estimates in Chart 3.2, page 30, the number of uninsured rose from about 25 million in 1977 to 37 million in 1988, and costs as a percentage of GNP rose from 8.5 percent to 11.3 percent.

Reasons for Noncoverage

Although Medicaid, which was enacted in 1965 along with Medicare, is a program aimed primarily at the poor, it has always failed to cover a substantial proportion of the families and individuals who are poor. In recent years, Medicaid coverage has been on a roller coaster. About a million working mothers and their children were removed from the rolls in the early 1980s. More recently, congressional action has increased coverage, with further expansion to take place in the coming years. Eventually, all poor children 18 years and under are slated to be covered, but many poor adults, both working and nonworking, are not. Blocking many from coverage are eligibility levels set below poverty in most states as well as

Chart 3.2: U.S. Health Care Costs and the Uninsured, 1977-88

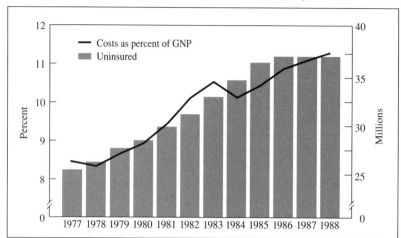

Sources: Costs—*Health Care Financing Review,* Spring 1989, Vol. 10, No. 3. Uninsured—EBRI, *Uninsured in the United States: The Nonelderly Population without Health Insurance, 1988* (Washington, D.C., September 1990).

strict asset tests. Among the employed, the working poor are most likely to be in jobs without health care coverage and also ineligible for Medicaid.

The United States is the only industrialized country (again with the exception of South Africa) where loss of job means loss of health care protection as well. In countries with universal health care entitlement, there is no link between employment and health care coverage. In the United States, this has always been a serious problem for the unemployed. In recent years, displacement of workers from blue collar jobs, many of them union jobs with comprehensive health care coverage, has caused the ranks of the uninsured to swell. Some displaced workers have been unable to find jobs for long periods of time and have been uncovered during their unemployment. For many displaced workers as well as those entering or returning to the labor force, their only employment opportunities have been in the expanding service sector or in small businesses in which many firms do not offer health care coverage at all or offer very limited health care benefits. The result of recent labor market trends has thus been to expand noncoverage.

The problem has been compounded because some hospitals, faced with serious financial losses, have reduced or eliminated uncompensated care on which uncovered low income people have depended for necessary medical care. Poor people without Medicaid coverage have resorted to public hospitals, which have traditionally provided them with free care. But these hospitals are now so crowded and are facing such critical financial problems that they have been forced to close wings, eliminate critical services and turn away less seriously ill patients.

Another factor expanding noncoverage is the refusal of a number of insurers to cover employees in some firms because their work is considered hazardous, low paying or seasonal. Insurers may also turn away or charge unaffordable premiums to firms, especially small firms, from which the insurer anticipates higher than normal claims rates or administrative costs. Recent media reports note that many insurance carriers are denying health care coverage to a wide gamut of small businesses and professions.

Further, as the *New York Times* recently reported, the phenomenon of "job lock" is growing. Those in job lock are afraid of changing jobs because their medical history would probably keep them from being accepted by a new health plan in today's stringent insurance market. The *Times* mentioned cancer patients and others with chronic diseases as being the most vulnerable.

In a similar vein, insurance is denied to some people with chronic diseases based on pre-existing medical conditions such as diabetes, cancer, mental illness, and heart disease. Hence, people who transfer employment may find that their coverage in a prior job is denied in the new one. Some insurers are even excluding from group coverage employees whose costs are expected to be especially high — those with serious medical conditions or who have dependents with such problems.

Effects of Noncoverage

The high incidence of lack of medical care coverage takes its toll in a large number of unnecessary illnesses and deaths as well as in much preventable chronic disease and disability.

The penalties of noncoverage begin at birth, and they are disproportionately borne by the poor and racial minorities. Although the U.S. infant mortality rate has declined somewhat in recent years, it is still one of the highest among industrialized countries, ranking about twentieth in the world. In 1989, the rate for blacks, 17.9 per 1,000, was almost twice the 9.1 rate for whites. The recent modest overall improvement is attributed to high cost medical technology rather than to expansion of prenatal care.

According to a 1987 report of the Alan Guttmacher Institute, lack of insurance leaves more than 1.3 million women each year without adequate prenatal care, and 555,000 women give birth without health insurance protection. These situations result in life-long health, learning and societal consequences that are well documented. There are also major financial consequences. According to the Institute, in 1985 the typical cost of having an average baby was nearly $5,000 compared with about $27,000 for an extremely premature infant. The Institute also reported that about $2.0 billion out of $7.4 billion in annual hospital losses for uncompensated care can be attributed to unpaid maternity care.

Lack of adequate care, especially in the inner city, has contributed to the reappearance of diseases such as tuberculosis, measles (in a more deadly form than in the past), mumps, and whooping cough, thought to have been completely or virtually eradicated. Those with low income (and, as discussed, therefore less likely to have health care protection) suffer more chronic diseases and have higher death rates. Uninsured patients are likely to be sicker upon admission to the hospital than are insured patients and up to three times as likely to die in the hospital.

The gaps in the current health care system have been both exacerbated and highlighted by the AIDS epidemic. In critical ways, the needs of AIDS victims are at variance with the way health care in America is financed and delivered. As their physical condition deteriorates, AIDS patients eventually have to stop work; when they do, they lose any health care coverage they may have had through their jobs. The costs of their illness remain high for the rest of their lives, and virtually none of them can afford to meet the expenses. This has exacerbated the financial crises facing many hospitals, especially inner city hospitals that are most likely to give uncompensated care. It has also forced hospitals to try to shift the uncompensated care for AIDS patients to other payers.

The lack of health care coverage for large numbers of Americans is widely seen as a major defect in the current U.S. health care system. Our failure thus far to assure universal access to health care is regarded as not just unfair and harmful to those who are not protected but also as harmful to society and the economy. Although there is no consensus on how universal access to care is to be achieved, all proponents of health care reform include it as a major goal in their programs. So too does President Bush. In his 1991 State of the Union address, he said, "Good health care is every American's right." Thus far, however, the Administration has not announced any specific proposals for achieving this goal.

Chapter IV

Quality of Care

The triad of concerns in everyone's goals for health care reform are cost, access and quality. But while cost and access are measurable, quality is not. In fact, there are many ideas about how to define quality of care and how to achieve that quality.

There is increasing agreement that assessing the quality of care must be based on health outcomes. Thus, a committee of the Institute of Medicine has defined quality of care as "the degree to which health services for individuals and populations increase the likelihood of desired health outcomes and are consistent with current professional knowledge" (Institute of Medicine, 1990, p. 4). Inherent in this definition is the concept that some health services are appropriate and therefore contribute to desired health outcomes, but that others are ineffective or even harmful under particular circumstances or perhaps even invariably and therefore do not contribute to desired health outcomes. Some believe that as much as one-fourth of all medical care may be of the latter variety. Of course, the inappropriate care may entail as high a cost (or even higher) than the care that is beneficial. Hence, getting a handle on the quality of care may contribute not only to the well-being of patients but also to the restraint of health care costs. Efforts are beginning in the private sector to inject more accountability into health care programs. Eleven large companies along with their insurers are introducing questionnaires developed by medical authorities to find out specific results of medical treatment from employees. The large auto companies and the United Auto Workers are involved in somewhat similar programs with the HMOs they use.

Physician Practice Patterns

Most consumers recognize that the technical nature of medical care inevitably requires that physicians will continue to make the critical decisions and have the principal responsibility for medical care. But consumers are nevertheless increasingly inclined to question the appropriateness of their care in their relations with their doctors and in more extreme ways such as malpractice litigation. Consumers have also become increasingly concerned about whether cost containment, which in general terms they endorse, could compromise the quality of care for themselves and their families. It therefore becomes all the more essential to marry the two goals of cost containment and quality enhancement.

Both in local communities and at the national level, studies are being made of how medicine is practiced and whether guidelines can be developed to make it more effective and conceivably, though not necessarily in all instances, less costly. One potentially important development is a study jointly sponsored by the American Medical Association and a consortium of academic medical centers aimed at developing practice guidelines for a large number of medical procedures. The guidelines will be based on data accumulated and analyzed by expert physician panels from particular specialties. Along the same lines, Congress has requested guidelines for four procedures — cataract surgery, aortic aneurysm surgery, carotid endarterectomy, and coronary bypass — from the Department of Health and Human Services. Other procedures are likely to be studied in the future. All of these efforts are aimed at improving the quality of care that is given and at eliminating the large amount of costly and often harmful unnecessary tests, medications, hospitalization, and surgery.

Assessment of New Technology and Procedures

There is a rigorous procedure for the assessment of new drugs and medications. In fact, it is so painstaking and time-consuming that AIDS patients who are anxious to use any new drug that might be helpful have complained that for their needs the procedure should be streamlined. But there are no controls on the introduction of new medical technology and no assessment of its effectiveness before it is introduced. The new technology, in turn, results in new procedures utilizing the technology without any prior test of their effectiveness. Proliferation of new technologies with no prior assessment of effectiveness undermines the quality of care and is a major factor in medical cost inflation. Various groups have recommended that a mechanism comparable to the Food and Drug Administration's program for assessing new drugs be developed for new procedures, technology and equipment.

Unnecessary Surgery

Other developments in the medical field affect both the quality and the cost of care. Since 1970, the number of surgeons has nearly doubled. At the same time, new nonsurgical and medical procedures have been developed that replace surgery for some conditions. One result is that in just three years, from 1982 to 1985, the number of operations performed by the average general surgeon dropped by 25 percent. There is concern that with the number of surgeons expanding more rapidly than the amount of needed surgery, surgeons may be performing too few operations to maintain their proficiency and thus may be tempted to expand minor or marginal procedures to avoid reducing their incomes. Although there may be a surplus of physicians in suburban middle class areas, there is a need for more surgeons in rural areas and inner cities. A redistribution of surgeons might contribute to meeting all three goals — quality, cost and access.

Preventive Health

Another quality-related issue is preventive health. By and large, private insurance programs have traditionally not covered preventive health services such as immunizations, wellness programs and testing, and neither has Medicare. This practice is slowly changing. HMOs, which have traditionally covered preventive services as an integral part of their programs, have found that prevention not only averts serious disease but is also cost effective. This is one reason why HMOs have much lower hospitalization rates than conventional insurance. Now the insurance industry is beginning to try to integrate at least some preventive care into its programs.

Hospital Care

Since 1986, the Health Care Financing Administration has been publishing mortality data of hospitals and making it available to the general public. HCFA has emphasized that high mortality rates per se may not necessarily indicate poor quality of care because there might be extenuating circumstances such as a higher incidence of very sick patients. But a high mortality rate may be a signal for further investigation of the hospital's quality of care.

The Joint Council for the Accreditation of Health Organizations has instituted a program with the cooperation of its affiliated hospitals aimed at helping them to enhance the quality of their care on the basis of outcomes measurement. JCAHO expects that development of good performance-based indicators will result in prompt investigation to remedy problems and produce better patient outcomes.

Cost Containment and Quality

As mentioned, some consumers and providers have expressed the fear that certain types of cost containment measures could adversely affect the quality of care. For example, it has become common for insurers to require that individuals get prior approval before going into a hospital for nonemergency care. The doctor's decision must be confirmed by the authorized representative of the insurer. The question is whether hospital precertification and other utilization review measures such as monitoring hospital length of stay may compromise the quality of care. In 1989, the Institute of Medicine concluded that there was no documented information to imply that prior review programs were placing patient safety in jeopardy. The Institute also warned that "premature or misguided regulation could stifle worthwhile innovations" in utilization review. Nevertheless, just as it is important to monitor the quality and effectiveness of care, it is also important to monitor the impact of cost containment measures to assure that they are compatible with maintaining quality of care.

Ethical Questions

Very much related to the quality of care are questions concerning the ethics of medical care that have come to the fore. Doctors, hospitals and patients and their family members, as well as purchasers and insurers of care, are being called upon to make excruciating life-and-death decisions. The decisions are essentially whether and under what circumstances heroic medical treatment of critically ill patients should be withdrawn and the patient be permitted to die a "natural death." The issue arises for patients of all ages, but the argument has tended to focus on the beginning and end of life — aggressive treatment to save the lives of very premature infants and the use of highly technical equipment to prolong the life of very old people who are considered in a vegetative or brain-dead condition. In each case, the questions are asked whether the life-prolonging treatment is in the interest of the patient and even if it is, is it worth the very high cost of such treatment. Some, especially adherents to the "right-to-life" philosophy, say that regardless of cost or the patient's pain or discomfort, any available measure should always be used if it will help to prolong a life. Others believe that heroic measures to prolong life should be withdrawn if that is the wish of the patient or the patient's family if the patient is incompetent, or if there is no prospect that the patient can be restored to a reasonable living condition. Consistent with this attitude is the growing use of a "living will," which authorizes the withdrawal of treatment that artificially prolongs life.

Also consistent with the idea of natural death is the rapid development of hospices throughout the country. Originally a British innovation in medical care, hospices are used by patients who are expected to die within a few months. These patients are provided care that makes their last days as comfortable, painless and life-enriching as possible. By and large, both patients and their families have been satisfied with the care that hospices have provided.

The discussion of ethical issues thus far has been limited to more or less voluntary decisions of patients or their families to limit heroic care. Oregon, however, has introduced restrictions on the care given to its Medicaid patients in an effort to expand Medicaid coverage significantly by ranking various procedures and limiting coverage to preventive care and treatable life-threatening conditions. Some have criticized the Oregon plan as rationing imposed only on the poor who depend on Medicaid while no such limitations are placed on medical care for the rest of the population. Others maintain that only relatively low priority care would be eliminated for those already under Medicaid in return for spreading protection to those who heretofore have had no protection at all. Still others have suggested that a plan similar to Oregon's should be used in health care for all people as a way of curbing health care inflation.

Both proponents and adversaries of the idea that there are conditions under which treatment may be withdrawn or not given at all are mindful of the cost consequences. There is probably no medical care more expensive than the care given to dying patients or to premature infants. Therefore, the ethical question is inevitably bound up with questions of allocation of available medical resources and the establishment of priorities. It is sometimes forgotten that decisions are made every day by providers, insurers and purchasers of care about the allocation of available resources. To some extent, these decisions are made on the basis of severity of illness; to a considerable extent, they are based on the patient's ability to pay for the needed treatment.

Chapter V

Attitudes Toward the Health Care System

The American people have indicated in polls taken over a period of at least 35 years that they are sufficiently dissatisfied with the American health care system that they would favor a national health care program. If this position is true, why is the United States almost the only industrialized country in the world without a national health program?

One reason for the lack of success of proposals for a national health program may be that, when polled, the overwhelming majority of Americans say they favor a national program, yet they do not name health care at the top of their list of the most important issues facing the country. According to a 1990 Gallup poll, 72 percent of respondents said they favored a national health program, but only 14 percent considered health care one of the two most important problems confronting the country. A year later, however, as has been mentioned, a national poll showed that health care ranked with the economy as an issue of prime concern. It is important to consider the answers that people give to questions about the health care system as an indication of the policies and possible reforms they might support.

Views of the Public

More than people in other countries, Americans believe that fundamental change is needed in their country's health care system. In 1988, Louis Harris and Associates conducted a survey of people's attitudes toward their country's health care system in 10 industrialized countries (the United States, Canada, Britain, West Germany, France, the Netherlands, Sweden, Italy, Japan, and Australia). The United States was the only country in that list without some type of national health program. Eighty-nine percent of Americans said their nation's health care system needed fundamental reform compared with 42 percent of Canadians and 69 percent of British respondents. Americans registered the most dissatisfaction and Canadians the least. The difference between Americans and Canadians was even more marked when people in each country were asked whether they would prefer the health care system of the other country. Sixty-nine percent of Americans said they would prefer the Canadian system, while only 3 percent of Canadians would replace their system with the American approach.

What are some of the reasons that Americans seem to be so dissatisfied with the current health care system? One issue can be ruled out — the quality of care that Americans personally receive. According to the Harris poll, 93 percent consider their own care to be of good quality. But they are concerned about its cost. According to a 1988 Roper poll, 53 percent of the respondents thought the cost of health care was very unreasonable (25 percent) or somewhat unreasonable (28 percent). More than 75 percent believed that health care costs were rising faster than the general inflation rate, and 57 percent thought that such costs were rising much faster.

Another reason for dissatisfaction is insecurity about health insurance coverage. A 1990 *Los Angeles Times* poll revealed that a substantial percentage of those polled, though not a majority, registered insecurity about paying for needed medical care. Twenty-nine percent said they did not have enough insurance to cover a "major medical expense"; 25 percent said they did not have enough money to pay for routine family health care; and the same proportion said they had put off medical treatment because they thought it would cost too much.

This poll showed that Americans want their government to be more active in the health care field even if a financial burden falls on them. Nearly three-fourths stated that they favor (about one-half of these strongly) a national comprehensive plan even if this means an increase in their taxes (Chart 5.1, page 42).

Periodic polls over the years have found that a substantial majority of Americans favor universal health care coverage. In 1990, several polls found that nearly three-fourths favored some form of national health care program. One poll found that to achieve universal coverage, 46 percent said they wanted a public plan and 33 percent a mixed private and public plan. Under the latter, all employers would be required to provide health insurance for their employees, and a government plan would provide for those not employed. The indecision between these two approaches is reflected in the proposals that have been put forth by individuals and groups dedicated to that goal.

Management's Attitudes

A 1991 Gallup survey for the Robert Wood Johnson Foundation found that 91 percent of the chief executives of the nation's largest firms that were surveyed felt that a fundamental change or complete rebuilding of the health care system is needed. Seventy-three percent thought that the problems in the health care system could not be solved by companies working on their own, and a majority said that government intervention is necessary. Nevertheless, 75 percent favored keeping the present employment-based structure. Only 33 percent favored a government-run health care system, 9

Chart 5.1: A Poll on National Health Care

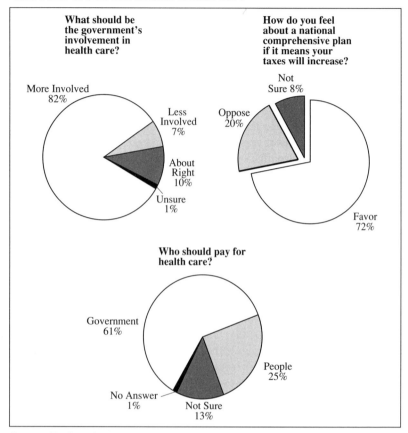

Source: Derived from a *Los Angeles Times* poll, 1990.

percent immediately and 24 percent for future consideration. A recent poll of corporate executives commissioned by the Metropolitan Life Insurance Company found that 53 percent might accept national health care if managed care failed to contain costs over the next few years. In the Gallup survey, 25 percent favored a government requirement for all employers to provide health benefits, and an additional 24 percent saw this as a future option. Just over 50 percent believed that there should be tax incentives to encourage small firms to provide health care coverage. Seventy-nine percent supported expanding public programs to cover the uninsured —

40 percent now and 39 percent as a future option. More than 60 percent wanted a single payment structure for hospitals and doctors binding on all payers, public and private.

Thus, an increasing number of employers (but undoubtedly still a minority) seem willing to consider some sort of approach, fostered or implemented by government, that would soon or in time result in universal health care, provided it included a strong element of cost containment. Employers who favor government action are divided, like other Americans, between a government-sponsored health insurance program and a program based on private insurance that would require all employers to provide a specified package of health care benefits (with a public program for the low income group and the unemployed).

Employers who favor a government program generally feel that only the government (most say the federal government) would be able to rationalize the current U.S. system. They call attention to the fact that the United States is virtually the only country in the world where the private sector rather than the government finances most health care of employees and their dependents. They also point to the absence of a national budget or expenditure target for health care, in contrast to such limitations in countries with national health care programs. They also believe that the rapidly inflating health care costs borne by U.S. employers place them in a disadvantageous position vis-a-vis their competitors in other countries. In those countries, health care costs are not the responsibility of employers but are spread over the entire population. Employers who are influenced by these considerations have, in some cases quite reluctantly, concluded that no one firm can deal with the problems of cost, access, quality, and competitiveness in U.S. health care and that, in fact, the country faces a national problem requiring a national solution.

Employers who provide health care coverage for their employees are especially concerned that they are in an unfair competitive situation with respect not just to foreign competitors but also to domestic competitors that do not provide health insurance or provide only very inadequate health insurance to their employees. To achieve a level playing field, these employers would require all employers to provide health care benefits.

Organized Labor's Position

Organized labor, as represented by the AFL-CIO, has made national health care reform its number one policy issue. For decades, the trade union movement has advocated adoption of national health insurance.

At the present time, organized labor's support for national health care reform is probably stronger than ever. Trade unions are alarmed that health care benefits that unions have won over a long period are being curtailed and are in serious jeopardy of being wiped out. Union leaders for the first time are seriously concerned about the imminent breakdown of the prevailing employment-based health insurance system. They are convinced that only a national health program will preserve workers' health care protection and also make health care a universal right, contain health care costs and assure the quality of health care.

Unions point to both the growing number of uncovered or inadequately covered workers and the shifting of costs from employers to employees (see Chart 2.2, page 13). Preserving health care benefits and the related question of who shall pay for escalating health care costs have become dominant issues in industrial disputes. Data compiled by the Service Employees International Union from a number of sources, including the Bureau of National Affairs and the U.S. Bureau of Labor Statistics, show that in 1986 health benefits were a prime factor in major work stoppages (1,000 or more workers) involving 18 percent of workers who went on strike. By 1989, that figure had climbed to an astounding 78 percent (Service Employees International Union, 1990).

In a number of major industries, generally after contentious negotiations or even strikes or lockouts involving health care benefits, the union and the employer have agreed to work together for national health care solutions. A typical example is an agreement in 1989 between the Bethlehem Steel Corporation and the United Steelworkers of America to set up a joint committee that would "seek to develop and support an appropriate national health policy which will assure essential care to all citizens, control health care costs and equitably distribute those costs across the various sectors of the economy." In a similar agreement between the American Telephone and Telegraph Company and its two principal unions, the Communications Workers of America and the International Brotherhood of Electrical Workers, it was declared that, "The Company and Unions agree that the problem of rising health care costs cannot be solved at the bargaining table and that the triple problem of access, cost and quality of health care are national problems requiring comprehensive national solutions." Labor and management have also agreed to work for national health care reform in the auto, bakery and men's clothing industries.

In 1990, the AFL-CIO launched a national health care campaign to inform union members, members of Congress and the public about the need for fundamental health care reform to deal with the systemic problems of access, cost and quality. The AFL-CIO conducted hearings in fall 1990 on health care in eight cities around the country, in which rank and file workers, union leaders, health care providers, insurers, and health care experts participated.

Chapter VI

Proposals for
Health Care Reform

There is a remarkable degree of consensus on the facts describing health care in America and on the shortcomings of the current system. With so much concern about health care focused on its undesirable aspects, it is not surprising that more thought is being given to health care reform than ever before.

Many of those engaged in formulating health care reform measures are paying greater attention than in the past to the experiences of other countries, particularly Canada. No one expects to adopt completely any foreign health care system, but Americans are increasingly aware of the differences between the U.S. system and those in other countries and are wondering if we can usefully adapt any of their features to improve our situation.

Consideration of health care reform is not limited to the national level. In fact, Hawaii and Massachusetts have already enacted universal programs, and other states are considering that route. In the 1970s and 1980s, some states adopted hospital rate-setting programs, measures to expand coverage of the noninsured, or both.

On another level, changes have been instituted that could have a bearing on national health care reform. Cost-containment measures have been adopted for Medicare, first affecting hospitals and later physicians' services, that some proponents of health care reform would incorporate in a national program that extended to the entire health care sector.

Perhaps of greatest interest are the proposals that have been offered and those that are in process for an American national health care program. A few proposals have been worked out in detail, but only the general principles of others have been agreed on. A number of them have been introduced as congressional bills.

Foreign Experience

Health care systems in industrialized countries generally fall into two categories, with both providing universal and comprehensive benefits.

- A *national health service*, with tax-financed government ownership of facilities and with doctors as public employees or on a kind of retainer and paid a fixed amount for each patient (capitation). This is the U.K. model.
- A *social insurance program*, with contributions paid either as taxes or premiums by some combination of employers, employees and general revenue and with providers in an independent status. (See Table 6.1, page 48, for selected features of programs in a number of major industrialized countries.)

Table 6.1: Structure and Financing of Selected Foreign Health Care Systems Compared with the U.S. System, 1988

	Financing Method	National Budget	Universal Coverage	Private Supplements	Paid by Government	Per Capita Cost
Canada	General Revenue/ Premiums	Total	Yes	Yes	76%	$1,370
France	Payroll Tax	Total	Yes	Yes	79	1,039
W. Germany	Payroll Tax	Total	Yes	Yes	78	1,031
Japan	Payroll Tax	Total	Yes	Yes	73	831
U.K.	General Revenue	Total	Yes	Yes	86	711
U.S.						
Under 65	Premiums	No	No	NA	41	1,926
Over 65	Payroll Tax/ Premiums	No	Yes	Yes		

Source: *Health Affairs,* Fall 1988, pp. 107 and 109. Reprinted with permission.

A principal difference in health care systems between the United States and most other countries is that the latter establish an annual national health care budget that sets a limitation on national health care expenditures. Another important difference is that other nations set uniform payment levels to providers prospectively in annual negotiations. Without a myriad of insurance organizations and no problems in determining coverage either of patients or services, the administrative costs of these health care systems are invariably lower than those of the United States.

In the United States, there is very little interest in trying to establish a national health service (or "socialized medicine" as it is sometimes called) like the United Kingdom's. Even those who favor that approach acknowledge that it has little or no chance of being adopted in this country. Therefore, attention has been directed to the social insurance models in other countries, especially in Canada, but also in Germany and perhaps in others. Here brief mention will be made of the Canadian and German systems.

Perhaps because of our proximity to Canada, much attention in recent years has been directed to its health care system. Some in the United States have advocated that we actually adopt a "Canadian-type system," and some proposals for an American national health program are said to be modeled on the Canadian system. Canada's universal health care system, like the United States' more limited program, is called "Medicare." It was implemented in two stages — hospitalization in 1956 and physicians' services in 1966. It combines national and provincial public financing with administration of payments to hospitals and physicians at the provincial level. Depending on the province, payments by the covered population are in the form of either premiums or taxes and are not employment-based.

It is important to point out that when Canadian Medicare got under way, only about one-third of Canadians had private health insurance. As the United States contemplates health care reform today, most Americans have health care coverage as an employment benefit. If the United States adopts the Canadian way of paying for health care, far more drastic changes will occur than Canada experienced in starting its system.

Other features of the Canadian system, however, are conceivably transferable across the border. Five basic principles underlie Canada's health care system: public administration, comprehensiveness, universal coverage, portability, and reasonable access. Minimum benefits applicable to all provinces are specified in the federal law. Expenditures are controlled through allocation of global budgets to hospitals and negotiation with physicians' organizations of fees and, in some provinces, volume of service. There is no participation of private insurers as either insurers or intermediaries. The ministry of health in each province funds the operating budgets of hospitals. Hospital capital investment is funded from various sources, the major one being the ministry; the investment must be approved by the ministry. Spending for physicians' services is restrained by fee schedules that the ministry negotiates with provincial medical associations. Because there is a centralized system with a single payer in each province, administrative costs are considerably lower than in the United States, as are total costs of the system. This is despite the fact that the Canadian system covers all Canadians, while the U.S. system fails to cover a significant number of Americans. Yet, the record of health care in Canada's less costly system is at least as good as the United States' record.

The German system is also a social insurance system, and it is also universal and comprehensive. However, it is quite different from Canada's system and in some ways more like that of the United States. Both financing and delivery of health care in Germany are pluralistic. Only a very small proportion of German health care spending is publicly funded. Most of it is provided and financed by over a thousand fiscally independent nonprofit sickness funds (we would call them health insurance funds), which are private but subject to requirements set forth in national legislation. An annual assembly, composed of all the major groups involved in health care in what is called the Concerted Action on Health Care, establishes economic guidelines for the health care system, including the overall expenditure growth rate. Although the assembly does not have mandatory powers, it has influenced annual fee negotiations and has helped to restrain German health care cost inflation.

The United States is not the only country considering reforms in its health care system. A number of European countries are discussing various changes that might make their universal systems more effective, including elements that would enhance regulated competition in health care. These developments should be watched to see if any of them might be incorporated, with whatever modification is appropriate, in the health care reform the United States undertakes.

While it is worthwhile to examine the experience of other countries as we in the United States contemplate health care reform, it is neither realistic nor appropriate for us to consider adopting the system of some other country, however successful it may be in the eyes of the citizens of the country. If the United States decides on major changes, we will inevitably develop our own system that will be different from those of other countries. We have no tradition of simply copying other countries' social programs. We have unique traditions, customs and government structure that will influence our decisions. Therefore, any changes we make will necessarily involve starting with what we have and deciding how much to change it and in what respects.

Health Care Reform in the States

Confronted with runaway health care costs and concerned that large numbers of their residents are unable to get needed care, some states are moving ahead to enact their own health care reforms without waiting for federal action. Hawaii and Massachusetts, as noted earlier, have enacted sweeping health care changes that aim at universal coverage. Other states are in various stages of considering similar legislation.

In 1974, Hawaii enacted a requirement that nearly all employers provide health care benefits, either fee-for-service or HMO, for their employees working at least 20 hours a week. Although dependent coverage is voluntary, the state health department has estimated that there is 95 percent coverage. To fill the remaining 5 percent gap, in 1990 Hawaii launched the State Health Insurance Program with emphasis on preventive and primary care. In this program, costs are shared between the state and individual on a sliding scale based on income.

The universal health insurance initiative in Massachusetts stems from its Health Security Act of 1988. All residents are to have access to affordable health care by 1993. Implementation of the 1988 legislation began with coverage through a state program for the unemployed and a requirement for full-time college and university students to purchase health insurance through their institution or a comparable plan. For coverage of workers and their families, Massachusetts has a "play or pay" requirement scheduled to go into effect in 1993. At that time, businesses with more than five employees will be required to pay a surcharge of 12 percent of each full-time employee's first $14,000 in wages into a health insurance trust fund up to a maximum of $1,680 per employee. Employers who provide at least the level of benefits the law requires can deduct the cost of such benefits from the surcharge. Employees of firms that do not provide coverage would be eligible on a sliding scale of payments in the state program. There is now some question whether the Massachusetts program will take effect. The governor is calling for repeal. Others would postpone until 1994 the requirement for employers to provide or pay for coverage.

Perhaps another 10 states are in various stages of developing legislation aimed at establishing universal coverage. Oregon will probably institute mandatory employer benefits in 1994, which will require employers to provide employee and dependent coverage or pay a tax. A companion measure sets up a state program to provide coverage to low income people not covered by employers or Medicaid. Other states in which legislation looking toward universal coverage has been introduced or proposed include Washington, California, Michigan, Missouri, Ohio, Oregon, Connecticut, Minnesota, and New York.

It is not clear how state action will affect the movement for national health care reform. Some argue that if a significant number of states enact universal coverage, it will relieve pressure on the federal government for a national program. Others feel that if a few more states, particularly large states, adopt universal coverage, national action for universal coverage is more likely.

Medicare Features Applicable to Health Care Reform

Any national health care program will have to limit the hospital costs the program will pay for. Medicare Part A has a prospective system for paying hospitals for inpatient stays that is based on the average cost for several hundred medical conditions called "diagnostic-related groups." If the hospital can meet Medicare requirements at less than Medicare's DRG rate, it pockets the difference. If it exceeds the DRG rate, it has to absorb the additional amount. This puts pressure on hospitals to reduce their costs and particularly the length of stay of Medicare patients. In 1991, the Health Care Financing Administration, which administers Medicare, announced a similar system for hospital outpatient care. Some proponents of national health care reform would incorporate the DRG system of hospital cost regulation in their programs. Others favor the system of negotiating hospital budgets used in Canada. Still others favor hospital rate-setting along the lines of state programs. In any case, the introduction of hospital cost regulation in Medicare has shown that some form of limitation of hospital costs in a national program is feasible and, on the whole, acceptable.

A number of new provisions aimed at reducing costs and enhancing quality of physician care under Medicare Part B are also suggested for inclusion in national health reform proposals. The most radical feature calls for annual "volume performance standards" for Part B services, the term used for what are really total national expenditure targets. Based on recommendations of the Physician Payment Review Commission and the Secretary of Health and Human Services, each year Congress will set the percentage increase for Part B spending. If it is exceeded in one year, the excess will be reflected in lower fees paid to physicians in the following year. Advocates of various national health reform proposals have incorporated the concept in their programs and would extend it by establishing annual spending caps on all health care expenditures.

Medicare fees are to be paid according to a fee schedule based on the relative worth of physicians' services. The criteria used in working out the relative value scale on which the fee schedule will be based were developed through cooperative efforts of physicians' groups, health care experts and the federal government. It is expected that in the future Medicare will be paying highly specialized physicians relatively less and those providing primary care and what has come to be called "cognitive" care relatively more. The fees will also determine the amount that doctors will be permitted to charge Medicare patients. Beginning in 1991, the charges may not be more than 25 percent over the fee schedule amount, in 1992, 20 percent, and thereafter 15 percent. Organizations of the elderly have long advocated "mandatory assignment" that would permit doctors to charge only the Medicare-approved fee.

One other innovation in Part B is the development of physician practice patterns. These are guidelines for medical procedures and treatment that are being developed by groups of physicians based on what they consider to be the most appropriate medical care. It is hoped that when these guidelines are fully developed, they will reduce unneeded care and, at the same time, improve the quality of care.

All the features that have been introduced in Medicare have a relevancy for national health care reform. Indeed, if the United States does establish a national health program, Medicare may well have paved the way by demonstrating the practicability and acceptance of features that would have to be incorporated in any viable national health program.

Proposals for National Programs

In recent years, a number of proposals for national health programs have been advanced, and others are in various stages of development. Sensitive to the widespread lack of health care coverage, the advocates of each of these proposals maintain that their plan will expand access to care and, at least eventually, achieve universal coverage. They also assert that their plans will moderate health care cost inflation and improve the quality of care.

Most of the proposals involve the following two approaches:
• mandatory employer coverage combined with a public plan covering a significant proportion of the population, including some who are not low income or poor;
• a single federal or federal-state program.

However, some proposals involve neither, and they will be described first.

Limited proposals. In February 1990, the Health Insurance Association of America announced its "Strategy for Containing Health Care Costs." Although HIAA's recommendations focused mainly on costs, they also included recommendations to expand coverage in various ways and to achieve quality improvement. Together these recommendations did not constitute a national health program, nor was this HIAA's intention. HIAA stressed the desirability of retaining a role for private insurance. There is no indication that if all of HIAA's recommendations were followed, the result would be universal coverage. However, to achieve broader coverage, HIAA has recommended establishment of state risk pools financed by state general revenues or other broad-based financing. These funds would permit small employers, people with severe health problems and other individuals to purchase private health insurance at lower rates than they could otherwise obtain. HIAA also recommends that Medicaid cover all people below the federal poverty level. It has a number of recommendations relating to cost containment, but particularly stresses the greater use of managed care.

In fact, in its public statements, HIAA has offered managed care as an alternative to a national health program. Others would incorporate expansion of managed care and some of the other HIAA recommendations in their broader national health reform proposals. Federal legislation has recently been introduced somewhat along the lines of HIAA's recommendations that would require, in one bill, employers with 3 to 25 employees and, in another, insurers selling to such firms to offer a basic health insurance package for voluntary purchase by employees. Although some 20 million employees and their dependents would be eligible to buy the insurance, undoubtedly far fewer would do so.

The Heritage Foundation has proposed a program that is explicitly intended to "give all Americans access to adequate health care services." The Foundation defines such services as including only catastrophic health care and would require individuals, not employers, to purchase the insurance. Low income workers would receive subsidies to help them buy the insurance. Medicaid would be continued for the poor, although states could provide narrower benefits than are now required. Medicare would also be continued, but mainly for catastrophic illness. A means-tested long-term care program would be established to be supplemented by private funds in various forms. Thus far, the Heritage program has received very little support. Most people would not be content with only catastrophic coverage. Moreover, most are reasonably satisfied with employment-based coverage and would not want to exchange it for a system based on individual insurance. In addition, it is hard to see how the Heritage proposal would not greatly add to already excessive health care administrative costs.

The Bush Administration appears to oppose both mandatory employer coverage and any new public program. Though there has as yet been no official pronouncement from the Administration, Secretary of Health and Human Services Louis W. Sullivan has said that he will not recommend to the President federally funded national health insurance because "the belief that putting an insurance card in every pocket will cure all our health care ills is false prophecy from those preaching easy solutions." Sullivan has pointed to problems such as poor diets, the spread of AIDS and substance abuse, the lack of health care facilities and health professionals especially in the inner cities, and the financial problems faced by some hospitals, all of which would not be automatically solved by national health insurance. Most proponents of universal health care programs would agree with him, but they would also maintain that assuring access to care for all Americans would mitigate such problems even if additional targeted action would still be required.

Comprehensive proposals. A number of proposals have been advanced or are being developed that would require all employers to provide, or in some way pay for, health insurance for their employees. These are the play or pay plans briefly discussed above. Because a majority of the uninsured are employees or their dependents, such a requirement would by itself constitute a long step toward assuring universal access. But there would still be uninsured people not holding jobs. To insure most of the remaining uncovered, advocates of mandating employer coverage recommend Medicaid expansion or some other public program.

Like the state programs in Hawaii, Massachusetts and Oregon, most of the employer mandate proposals would require employers who do not wish to provide health insurance for their employees at a specific minimum level of coverage to purchase it from Medicaid, or other public program, or to pay into a public fund that would finance care for employees not covered by employer plans. Among the proposals that fit this pattern are those of the National Leadership Commission (now the National Leadership Coalition) on Health Care Reform, the United States Bipartisan Commission on Comprehensive Health Care (the Pepper Commission) and the AFL-CIO. The American Medical Association favors an employer mandate and broader Medicaid coverage, but it has not recommended the play or pay approach. In addition to their coverage provisions, most of these proposals also include measures aimed at cost containment and quality enhancement.

In June 1991, a number of Senate Democratic leaders in health care (Senate Majority Leader George J. Mitchell and Senators Edward M. Kennedy, Donald W. Riegle, Jr., and John D. Rockefeller IV) introduced a bill based on the play or pay approach. It would require employers to provide at least a specified health care package for their employees or to pay a payroll tax to finance coverage for their employees through a new public program. The public program would also cover the poor, replacing Medicaid, and other uninsured people.

All of the proposals mentioned above are predicated on the continuance of private health insurance in an employment-based system, although most of them would assign a large supplementary role to a parallel public system serving certain individuals and groups. Another group of proposals would either exclude private insurers altogether or assign them only the intermediary administrative role they have in Medicare; that is, they would be administrative agents of a publicly funded program. Again, the proposals in this category are not all alike. However, generally they involve what is called a single payer (that is, payer of providers), a state or federal governmental or quasi-governmental organization, with payments to that payer in the form of either premiums or taxes by employers, employees and others. Health care for the poor would be subsidized, and those not employed would pay on some basis that is income related.

Proposals along these lines have been offered by Representatives Fortney ("Pete") Stark and Marty Russo as well as other members of Congress, Physicians for a National Health Program, the Health Security Action Council, and the National Association of Social Workers. These proposals, like those based on the employer mandate approach, include various cost-containment and quality improvement features, emphasize expanding managed care, and are often referred to as "Canadian-type."

In February 1991, the AFL-CIO Executive Council in a unanimous statement called for expeditious enactment of federal legislation for national health care reform. While maintaining its traditional goal of a national social insurance program for universal access to health care, as an immediate measure it set forth a play or pay plan. The AFL-CIO urged that all employers, including the federal government, be required to contribute fairly toward the cost of care. Specifically, employers could meet the requirement either by providing health care benefits themselves or by paying into a fund that would provide health care benefits for their employees. The latter would be a "national social insurance program" that would include employees not covered by employer benefits, as well as the unemployed and others not in the labor force, and would incorporate Medicare and Medicaid. The AFL-CIO program also calls for:

- a national cost-containment program that includes a cap on total health care expenditures, a capital budget and all-payer uniform reimbursement of rates negotiated by a federal authority with hospitals, doctors and other providers;
- a national commission of consumer, labor, management, government, and providers to administer the program;

• a core package of benefits with voluntary supplemental benefits;
• progressive and equitable financing;
• streamlined administration with involvement of intermediaries that, among other responsibilities, would have to assure that no one would be denied coverage;
• dropping the Medicare eligibility age from 65 to 60;
• various measures to improve quality and encourage avoidance of unnecessary tests and procedures and, as a related matter, developing a better system for handling malpractice disputes; and
• developing a strategy for universal access to long-term care, including home health care.

President Lane Kirkland of the AFL-CIO has emphasized that his organization is "not committed to any rigid, single plan" and is prepared to negotiate the details of a plan that will garner the broadest possible support.

Issues in National Health Care Reform

Coverage. Concern about escalating health care costs is the engine driving health care reform. But deprivation of access to care and its devastating consequences for millions of Americans deeply trouble the consciences of more fortunate Americans. This is why access to health care has come to be widely recognized as a fundamental right. It is worthwhile, then, to consider what would and what would not result in universal coverage.

Clearly, simply requiring employers to provide health insurance for their employees would not assure universal coverage; the nonemployed must also be assured of access to affordable health care. But there is a further question. Should the United States break the link between employment and the right to obtain health care as other countries have done? Payments for health care could be required of employers and employees as well as others, but failure to discharge such financial obligations would not affect anyone's eligibility to obtain needed health care to the extent the national legislation provides. There might be other penalties for not paying health care taxes or premiums but not denial of health care. Denial of health care as a penalty for failing to meet financial obligations affects dependents, especially children, who have no responsibility in the matter. Also especially affected are low income people who might be unable to meet their financial obligations even if these were reduced, but who are also most likely to need care.

Staging. Another issue is whether universal coverage should be achieved in stages or all at once. There are some who feel that, just as Medicare began with the elderly and then was extended to the severely disabled, the next group to be universally covered should be children. Indeed, recent expansion measures under Medicaid have aimed at complete coverage of poor children in the foreseeable future. But to extend universal coverage to all children while denying it to older family members would create both social and administrative difficulties. It seems very unlikely that legislation would be enacted requiring employers to provide coverage for their employees' children but not the employees themselves. Thus, the only way to assure access to health care for all children would be through a public plan. Once children, the elderly, the disabled, and the poor are covered under one or more public plans, it is likely that the next step would be to extend public coverage to employees too so that families would not be split between employer-based plans and the public plan or plans.

Other staging issues relate to how much time should be given to firms not now providing health insurance to their employees to purchase insurance or contribute to an alternative public plan. Also, particularly with respect to small firms, there is the question of whether they should receive a tax credit or subsidy when they begin to provide coverage or contribute to the public plan, and if so, for how long. The Pepper Commission plan would be staged in over a seven-year period, depending on the size of firm, with a subsidy for newly covered firms phased out over the same period.

Public versus private. The issue is not really public versus private because approximately 30 percent of current health care spending is already public. Rather, the question is whether there should be a public plan in addition to Medicare and Medicaid (or subsuming Medicare, Medicaid or both, as the AFL-CIO has proposed) that supplements private coverage or, alternatively, one which entirely replaces it, as a number of groups have recommended. The distinction between these two approaches may not be as sharp as it seems. Advocates of the play or pay approach would require employers to cover their employees. But they also recognize that some employers would choose to cover their employees under an alternative public plan.

On the other hand, it would be possible to have a program based mainly on a public plan but permitting employers meeting specified standards and requirements relating to access, cost and quality to opt out of the public plan in favor of private coverage. Again, it is hard to predict how many employers would choose this route. But assuming the characteristics of the two alternatives, and they are not altogether improbable, a private-public plan might not be so different from a public-private plan. Both would involve a large proportion of the population under private coverage and a large proportion under public coverage. However, there might be other important differences, including the proportions that would be privately and publicly funded and the amount that would show up in the federal (or state in a federal-state program like Canada's) budget. Also, even the public plan does not have to be totally public. Along the lines of the AFL-CIO proposal, that plan might follow the Medicare plan of using private insurance firms to administer the program. Their role might be similar to what they are already doing in employer-sponsored plans that are self-insured.

If the program includes a public plan, it is essential that such a plan not turn into the second-class plan that Medicaid has become. A unified reimbursement system would discourage providers from either avoiding the public plan or providing second-rate service to its participants. Also, inclusion of large numbers of nonpoor people under the public plan would mean that it should not be stigmatized as a poor person's or welfare plan as Medicaid has been. Nevertheless, strong efforts would have to be made to ensure that the public plan provides affordable access, and not just eligibility, as well as high quality standards.

Financing. Traditionally, benefit programs in the United States, both public and private, have been employment-based. Whether they have been privately insured like health care and pensions or publicly financed like social security and unemployment compensation, they have been largely funded by employer and, in some programs, employee payments in the form of either premiums or payroll taxes. This has proved to be an acceptable way of financing these social protections and, therefore, there is no reason for shifting to a program based on individual financing of either private insurance or public expenditures for health care. Sometimes the Canadian experience, which does involve individual premiums or taxes, is cited, but the situation in the United States is now quite different from Canada's when it began its Medicare program. Retaining employment-based financing would tend to minimize disruption and dissatisfaction in the transition to national health care reform.

A second issue relating to financing is how the financial burden of the cost of health care should be spread. There are several aspects of this question, and all relate to the extent to which health care funding can be geared to what the various elements in society can afford. Of course, effective health care cost containment will lighten the total financial burden, but it will not eliminate the question of how it should be distributed. The present system of financing health care is regressive in that small employers and their employees and individuals not only pay a higher percentage of income or payroll than large firms and their workers but are also likely to pay higher dollar amounts. At one time, so-called community rating was widespread in the United States. Under community rating, insurance rates are set on the same terms to all purchasers regardless of factors such as pre-existing conditions, claims experience, demographic characteristics, or size of firm. Community rating tends to hold down premium levels for higher risk groups. The Pepper Commission and the AFL-CIO would require community rating. The National Leadership Commission on Health Care recommended a play or pay plan in which employers choosing to pay into a public fund would be liable for a percentage of payroll and employees for a percentage of wages. The commission's plan therefore would offer a progressive financing alternative to employers wanting to take advantage of it. If a program is adopted that includes private and public components, reasonably equitable financing can be achieved by requiring community rating in the private component and relating premiums in the public component to payroll or income.

A major point of contention between unions and employers has been the shifting of costs from employers to employees. This raises the question of cost sharing. Sometimes the issue is posed as to whether there should be "first dollar coverage" or whether deductibles, co-payments or co-insurance and premium sharing should be permitted. Canadian law prohibits the imposition of payments on patients at the point of service. Canadians pay for their health care in taxes and premiums, not when they are sick and need care. They have first dollar coverage guaranteed by law. But first dollar coverage has almost disappeared in the United States. Except for HMO members and Medicaid participants who generally pay very little or nothing in deductibles, co-payments or co-insurance, nearly everyone else is liable for cost-sharing payments. It is unlikely that cost sharing would be eliminated in national health care reform. Most of the proposals offered thus far permit cost sharing but with limits on the level of deductibles, co-insurance or co-payments and shared premiums. The proposals also set a maximum for total out-of-pocket costs to be paid by an individual or family.

The argument for cost sharing is not just that insured persons should pay for part of the cost of the care that they and their families receive, but that requiring them to pay part of the cost encourages consumers to seek and use health care more judiciously. One way of doing this is to place less onerous cost-sharing requirements on those who elect to obtain their care in managed care systems that are considered more cost effective. Those who look with disfavor on cost sharing believe that it is likely to discourage preventive care and early treatment, with care being given at a later stage, resulting in both more suffering and higher cost. Opponents also point to the fact that as few as 10 percent of patients, generally the sickest ones, incur perhaps as high as 75 percent of total medical care costs. Moreover, especially if these high users have chronic conditions, they are likely to have reduced incomes resulting from their inability to work. Some national health care reform proposals, such as that of the National Leadership Commission on Health Care, provide for income-related cost sharing. This might be a more equitable approach, but it is also likely to engender higher administrative costs.

It is unlikely that cost sharing will be eliminated in the United States in the foreseeable future. As proposals are developed for health care reform, however, it is important that whatever cost-sharing payments are included should not be so burdensome as to discourage or bar needed care. Unfortunately, it is not easy to determine at what level of cost sharing that will occur because it depends very much on factors such as income, health condition and physical access to care.

Cost containment. It is most unlikely that any national health care reform program will be adopted unless strong cost-containment features are built into its structure. A consensus is beginning to develop on what these should be, although not all groups that have made, or are developing, proposals agree on all of them. Most are already being applied or are about to be applied in either public or private programs or both. Measures relating to cost are closely related to access and quality, and most observers of the health care scene agree that not only does cost containment not have to lessen access and quality but that it is essential to enhancing them.

The following are some of the main elements of a cost-containment policy.

- *A national budget for health care.* Countries like Canada and Germany have found that an annual national budget, which if exceeded in one year results in lower payments to providers in the following year, is perhaps the strongest available tool for achieving cost containment. The U.S. system has this tool now, but it is limited to physicians' services under Medicare Part B. While the National Leadership Commission on Health Care did not endorse the concept, it referred to it favorably. The AFL-CIO and other groups have recommended it outright. Inclusion of a cap on health care spending in national health care reform might be the best guarantee that expenditures will not be open-ended.

Recently, Comptroller General Charles A. Bowsher in testimony presented to the House Ways and Means Committee said that the United States "must move from incremental cost-cutting initiatives to reforms that encompass the entire U.S. health care system." He then went on to recommend that "we should cap total expenditures for major categories of providers and services, including physicians, hospitals and new technology." He said that maximum health expenditures could be adjusted each year so that if spending for a particular category exceeded its target in one year, it would be reduced the following year.

- *Negotiation of uniform payments to hospitals, doctors and other providers to be used by all payers.* This will require a decision as to what systems are effective in determining payments to hospitals and how they should be established or negotiated. It will also require negotiation of fee schedules with the representatives of physicians. Further, it is important that the payment systems be flexible enough to be appropriate for and encourage participation in HMOs and other forms of managed care.

- *Controls on capital expenditures.* The United States has the most advanced medical equipment in the world. Progress in medical technology should be encouraged. Nevertheless, we need to ensure that our medical plant and equipment are used in the most effective manner. This calls for assessment of new technology and procedures similar to the assessment system we already have for new drugs as well as controls on the proliferation of medical equipment. This would ensure that new technology and procedures are used in the most cost effective manner, that unnecessary duplication is eliminated and that quality is maintained.

- *Physician practice patterns.* Because decisions of physicians largely determine the cost and quality of medical care, it is important that guidelines be developed to assist physicians in their practice. This will not only enhance the quality of their care, but it will also discourage unnecessary tests and procedures.

- *Malpractice reform that is fair to both patients and providers.* There is probably less of a consensus on what ought to be done in this area than in any other affecting health care costs. But the experience of other countries with considerably lower malpractice insurance rates may help the United States to develop ways of dealing with this problem.

Quality. The great variation in the way physicians practice medicine affects its cost and also reflects differences in quality of care. The underlying problem seems to be an inadequate scientific base for the decisions that doctors and other providers have to make every day. Therefore, the development of systems for measuring outcomes of care is essential to quality enhancement. This will require building a national data base on the cost and quality of care. It is encouraging that a number of national health care reform proposals stress the importance of incorporating a quality improvement initiative and allocating dedicated funds for that purpose. Some aspects of quality enhancement are inevitably technical and, therefore, must be left to physicians and others with the appropriate scientific knowledge. It is, however, important that consumers and payers are also involved both in encouraging the quality improvement efforts of the professionals and in utilizing their own experience with the health care system as one important indication of medical outcomes.

Chapter VII

Long-Term Care

This report has focused primarily on the problems and issues involved in America's system for financing and delivering acute health care. However, it would not be complete if it were to ignore the problems and gaps in America's long-term care system on which chronically ill Americans of all ages depend.

Spending for Long-Term Care

There are two types of long-term care — nursing home care and home health care. In the United States, paid long-term care is overwhelmingly nursing home care. Home health care is largely unpaid care given by family members who are mostly women. Although most of paid long-term care is for nursing homes, more than twice as many in long-term care are at home than in nursing homes. A majority of the over-65 group are at home, and an overwhelming proportion of younger people receiving long-term care are at home.

About four-fifths of long-term care spending — about $50 billion a year — goes for nursing homes. Patients and their families pay for just over one-half of nursing home bills. Medicaid pays most of the rest (41 percent), with Medicare accounting for only 2 percent.

Nursing home expenditures have increased more than 10 times since 1970, and they have more than doubled in the past 10 years. According to a Brookings Institution study, if there were no change in public policy, nursing home expenditures could double again by the turn of the century and more than triple by 2020 (Rivlin and Wiener, 1988). Home care expenditures could also nearly triple by that year, but would still be dwarfed by spending for nursing home care.

Long-term care is not just a problem for the elderly. More than one-half of those receiving long-term care are under 65 (Chart 7.1, page 66). In addition, nonelderly care givers as well as the younger population, anticipating that some day they too will have a chronic condition requiring long-term care, could be greatly affected by how the United States decides to handle long-term care policy. Younger family members are also affected because the time and money they spend in caring for their elderly or disabled relatives may detract from their ability to meet their own needs and especially those of their children. Long-term care puts a tremendous financial and emotional burden on families, especially on adult women. Many of these women are trying to hold down full-time jobs while juggling their responsibilities for both old and young family members. Those in that

Chart 7.1: The Growing Burden of Long-Term Care: What We Spend on Nursing Homes

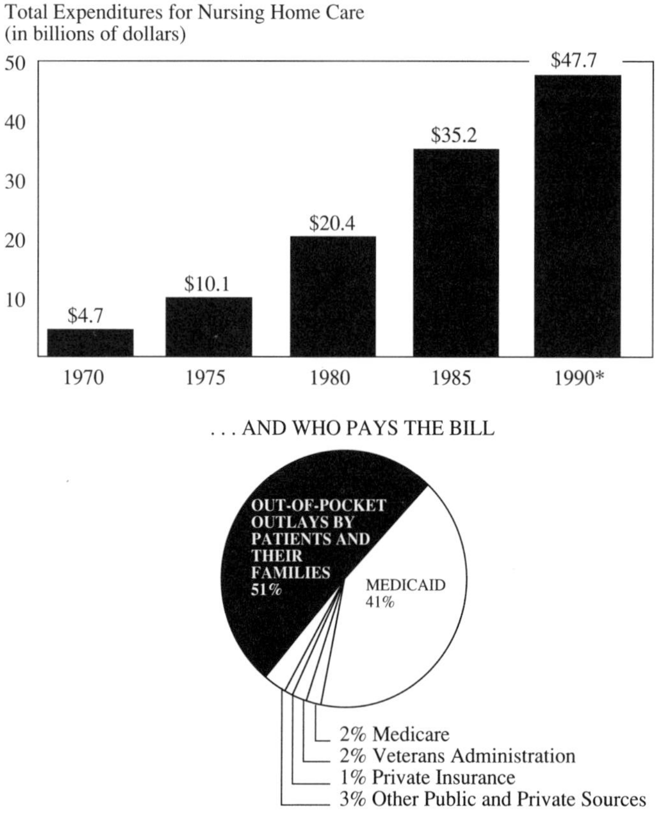

Total Expenditures for Nursing Home Care
(in billions of dollars)

1970	$4.7
1975	$10.1
1980	$20.4
1985	$35.2
1990*	$47.7

. . . AND WHO PAYS THE BILL

OUT-OF-POCKET OUTLAYS BY PATIENTS AND THEIR FAMILIES 51%
MEDICAID 41%
2% Medicare
2% Veterans Administration
1% Private Insurance
3% Other Public and Private Sources

* Estimate for 1990 based on $38.1 billion actual outlays for 1986 plus inflation at 5.8% per year.

Source: Robert M. Ball with Thomas N. Bethell, *Because We're All in This Together* (Washington, D.C.: Families U.S.A. Foundation, 1989), p. 15. Reprinted with permission.

precarious situation are often referred to as the "sandwich generation." Unfortunately, many of the elderly do not have family members on whom they can rely. A National Bureau of Economic Research study found that in Massachusetts, one-fifth of the elderly have no children and over one-half have no daughter (daughters do most of the unpaid care-giving) or have none living close enough to help them. The study also found that two-fifths of the elderly needing help with daily living activities live alone.

Although people of all ages may need long-term care, the elderly and especially the very old are far more likely to need long-term care than the younger population. A large proportion are likely to be in a nursing home at some time before their death. According to a 1991 study of the Agency for Health Care Policy Research, Department of Health and Human Services (HHS), it is anticipated that 43 percent of the approximately 2.2 million people who reached 65 in 1990 will eventually enter a nursing home, and 20 percent will spend at least five years in a nursing home. Nearly two-thirds of these elderly nursing home occupants will be women.

Staying in a nursing home is very expensive, and nursing home occupancy and costs have been rising quite rapidly. Total nursing home expenditures in 1989 were $48 billion. According to the HHS study, the annual cost of being in a nursing home averages about $25,000, far beyond the resources of elderly people whose primary income is from social security. Nearly all of the one-fifth of the elderly who will spend five years or more in a nursing home will exhaust their financial resources long before their stay is ended. They will then be eligible for Medicaid, which pays for more than 40 percent of nursing home care for those who are initially poor or who "spend down" to the Medicaid eligibility level. Both Medicare and private insurance pay for only a miniscule proportion of nursing home costs.

Most people with chronic health problems prefer to stay in their own homes for as long as possible and regard going to a nursing home as a last resort. It is then that they spend down to the Medicaid level and thereafter depend on Medicaid to defray the costs. In fact, the largest proportion of Medicaid spending is for nursing home care. This has distorted Medicaid's original purpose of providing acute care for needy families with children. Because nursing home proprietors often consider Medicaid payments inadequate, they frequently either refuse to admit Medicaid patients or provide them with inferior care.

While private long-term care insurance has increased rapidly in recent years, it still accounts for only a tiny percentage of long-term care. Although it may continue to expand, private long-term care insurance is not expected to finance a large proportion of long-term care in the future. Various studies have suggested a range of proportions that private insurance might eventually reach. Even an optimistic study, sponsored by the Health Insurance Association of America in 1991, found that more than one-half of the elderly cannot afford private insurance and that private insurance will never solve the problem. Other studies have reached even more pessimistic conclusions. While a very few firms have begun to offer various types of long-term care assistance to their employees, those that offer insurance require employees to pay the full premium cost, and others simply provide information on available resources.

Nursing Home versus Home Health Care

As previously stated, most paid long-term care is for nursing homes, with costs divided mainly between out-of-pocket payments and Medicaid. On the other hand, most home health care is unpaid and given by family care givers. There is great dissatisfaction with both. Nursing home care is very costly, and for most middle class families it requires eventual resort to Medicaid, a welfare program that is very distasteful to them. With the large proportion of women in the labor force, it is increasingly unrealistic to rely on unpaid family care givers for the bulk of home health care.

The heading of this section suggests that nursing home care and home health care are alternatives. At any one time, they may well be alternatives, but both will obviously continue to be needed. The policy questions are which is to be emphasized and how can it be done. Most advocates of proposals for improving long-term care have recommended that maximum reliance should be placed on home health care while recognizing that sooner or later many people will reach a stage of disability that requires them to enter a nursing home, perhaps for the rest of their lives. But, as discussed above, until that stage is reached, people prefer to remain in their own homes as long as they can. There is no doubt that even paid home health care, although not cheap, is less expensive than institutionalized care. This is why a number of long-term care proposals provide more generous benefits for home health care than for institutional care.

The concern about proposals involving new sources of payment for home health care is whether there will be a massive switch from unpaid to paid health care. Experience in a number of Canadian provinces that have introduced entitlement programs for long-term care, including community-based home health care, is that expenditures can be limited by conditioning decisions on eligibility through assessment of appropriate care by multidiscipline case management teams.

Long-Term Care Proposals

In recognition of unmet current needs and anticipated heightened requirements for long-term care, a number of proposals have been offered for national legislation. Reflecting the prevailing public view, all of these proposals involve a greater role for the federal government. In a recent Gallup poll, 72 percent of the respondents said that long-term care of the elderly should be financed by the federal government even if it requires a tax increase. A majority also said that they would be willing to purchase private insurance. In both alternatives, the amount they would be willing to pay for taxes or premiums would be far less than what would be required for adequate protection.

Long-term care spending today involves a public-private partnership, and most of the current proposals would continue that sharing of responsibility but with an altered distribution of public and private spending. Some proposals primarily involve incentives for expanding private insurance, while others focus on new forms of public financing for both home and nursing home care.

Expanding private coverage. Some proposals would try to expand private insurance and make it more affordable by providing tax advantages to purchasers in the form of either tax-exempt savings accounts (similar to individual retirement accounts) or a tax credit or deduction from taxable income to offset the cost of insurance premiums. Because only relatively high income people could afford the insurance even with the preferential tax treatment, the subsidy involved would go to those least needing it. It would not at all help those with limited resources who could not afford to purchase the insurance but would nevertheless pay for it in their own taxes. Moreover, unless prohibited from doing so, private insurers would continue to use underwriting and benefit criteria that would bar even some who could afford the insurance. In addition, the costs would continue to be inflated by the marketing and sales costs that private insurance entails.

These problems lead to the conclusion that reliance should not be placed exclusively on private insurance to achieve adequate long-term care for Americans. Nevertheless, there seems to be no doubt that even if there is an increase in the public role, private insurance will be an important element in long-term care. This is reflected in most of the proposals that involve expanding public financing of long-term care.

69

Proposals involving an increased public role. A number of bills have been introduced in recent years that provide for public financing of long-term care. A distinction is made between home and nursing home care, with more restrictive financing for the latter. The proposals provide for either back-end or front-end financing for nursing home care, with or without co-insurance. A bill introduced by Senator George J. Mitchell, for example, provides for community-based home care as soon as a certain stage of functional dependency is reached, but nursing home coverage would not be met for another two years.

Other proposals call for a reverse procedure. For example, the Pepper Commission proposal makes all severely disabled people eligible for a range of community and home care benefits. Federally financed nursing home care would be available universally only for three months with 20 percent co-insurance, except for those with incomes below twice the federal poverty level. After the three-month period, there would be joint federal-state financial responsibility, with patient payments related to assets and income. The program would be implemented in stages. The commission expected gaps to be filled by private insurance and, to encourage its development, the commission recommended favorable tax treatment comparable to what already applies to private health insurance for acute care.

The Pepper Commission estimated the cost of its long-term care program after full implementation at about $43 billion a year. Although it recommended no specific revenue sources, it laid down three principles for financing its proposal:
  • the tax package should be progressive;
  • the tax burden should fall on people of all ages; and
  • revenues should keep up with expanding needs.

Estimated costs for other proposals range from approximately $20 billion to $45 billion.

Chapter VIII

Conclusions

This study has sought to analyze the U.S. health care system and to set forth some of the ideas that have been put forward to reform it. There is no question that there is a greater desire for far-reaching changes in the way health care is financed and delivered than ever before. Also, there is more discussion of alternative solutions and more effort to bring together representatives of various groups. The goal is to develop a health care system that makes quality, affordable care available to all.

A number of proposals have been presented for achieving this goal, and others can be anticipated in the coming months. What can be said now about the prospects for national health care reform? If it is to come, what shape should it take?

Before trying to answer these questions, a caveat is in order. Despite the best intentions of many individuals and groups, it is far too soon to be sure that America will see far-reaching health care reform. There are large obstacles to its fruition. For some years, the governance of the country has been divided with a Republican President and a Democratic Congress. That will, of course, continue until 1993 and possibly beyond. It is difficult to launch major social initiatives when there is a divided government. Another negative factor is the nation's fiscal crisis. Any program that will bring about universal coverage will have to make care available to many people who cannot afford to pay for it. Therefore, even a program that relies primarily on private funding will inevitably require government expenditures above the current level, at least in its early stages. With the current tremendous budget deficit, there is great reluctance to add to government spending for domestic programs or to levy the taxes necessary to pay for them. Whether people who express a desire for health care reform will also support an adequate means of paying for it remains to be seen.

Despite these possible barriers to early action, much thought continues to be given to formulating recommendations for health care reform that can win broad enough support to have a reasonable chance of adoption. Aside from all the discussion and effort that is taking place at the national level, progress has been made in a number of states to develop comprehensive and universal state programs.

A year ago, it would have been foolhardy to try to suggest what might be the outlines of a program that might be offered as an alternative to the current system. Now the picture is beginning to be a little less murky. Although there are major differences among the various proposals, there is some evidence that one approach that is rooted in American experience is beginning to be favored by many, but not all, of those who are actively promoting health care reform. This is the approach, often referred to as play or pay, that is based on the requirement that employers either provide health care benefits for their employees or pay into a public fund that will do so.

In a number of groups, government and nongovernment, the details of specific proposals based on the play or pay approach are being hammered out. Participants in these groups are trying to agree on specific responses to many of the issues set forth earlier. It is not the purpose of this report to duplicate what they are doing, nor is it possible at this stage to predict the exact contours of the proposals that will be put forth. It is possible, however, to suggest the goals that these proposals must achieve if they are to deal with the major defects in the current U.S. health care system. The members of the Committee on New American Realities — leaders of business, labor, agriculture, and academic institutions — endorse the following goals as essential elements of national health care reform.

Universal coverage. If the program does not achieve universal coverage all at once, it should have a specific timetable for doing so within a few years. The uninsured can be divided into two main categories — the employed and the nonemployed. The program should include specific measures for covering both groups. In a play or pay type of program, the employed should be covered with a requirement that employers either provide the statutory benefit level or buy into a public program that will cover the firm's employees. The nonemployed will presumably also be covered by the same public plan. Depending on the income of nonemployed participants, part or all of the costs of their health care will have to be defrayed by public funds, either federal or some combination of federal and state.

A basic level of comprehensive benefits. For benefits to be comprehensive, they should include, at the very least, preventive care, necessary medical treatment in all appropriate settings, hospitalization, and long-term care in the patient's home and in a nursing home. There is bound to be discussion either before or after the program is launched about inclusion of other types of care — mental health, substance abuse, vision, dental, chiropractic, and perhaps other services. The issue to be resolved is what should be the scope of the minimum program available to all and what should be left to supplemental benefits that remain voluntary and, in unionized firms, subject to collective bargaining.

Built-in cost controls. It is generally recognized that no health care reform proposal can garner political support unless it has strong cost control components. High on the list of such controls is a national cap on health care expenditures that, it is anticipated, would provide the ultimate discipline for avoiding excessive health care spending. Subsidiary to this global spending limitation would be a number of other measures that would make its achievement feasible. These would include fee schedules, a system for determining hospital reimbursement, encouragement of managed care, medical technology assessment, controls on capital expenditures, negotiation of uniform payments to providers, and specific ways of minimizing administrative costs.

Improvements in the quality of care. Various ways of trying to achieve this goal have been discussed earlier and will not be repeated here. They should be incorporated in the program. To make certain that more than just lip-service is given to this goal, it is essential that an administrative unit or a commission — or preferably both — be established and charged with the responsibility of enhancing quality in every aspect of health care. To assure that this can be done, dedicated funds should be set aside. Relative to total health care costs, the amount would not have to be large and, in fact, because quality care should also be cost effective, it may in the long run involve very little, if any, additional spending. But a specific focus on quality is essential not only to assure that people get the right treatment but also to assure support for the program from both patients and providers.

Long-term care. National health care reform will not be complete without a long-term care component. Although its benefits can be expected to go primarily to the elderly, it should be available to people of all ages who meet its requirements as to functional impairment. It should be comprehensive, which means that it should include community-based home care and nursing home care. To reduce the cost and improve the quality of long-term care, case management should be an important feature of the program. Some have advocated that long-term care should be financed entirely from public sources, either as a part of Medicare and financed by increased payroll taxes or from general revenue. Others have suggested that with financial incentives, private insurance can do the job. Complete reliance on either public financing or private insurance is unlikely to meet long-term care needs. Instead, if comprehensive long-term care is to be achieved, some combination of public and private financing will probably be necessary. Whatever the specific financing measures, they should provide an adequate level of care to all recipients at costs they can afford. Since the aging of the population will expand needs, it is important that arrangements are made from the start for the program to expand commensurate with the growing requirements.

Affordable, adequate and equitable financing. Perhaps this is the most difficult goal, but its achievement is absolutely necessary if there is to be genuine national health care reform to correct the defects in the current health care system. Henry Aaron of the Brookings Institution has estimated that universal access to health care could be achieved with roughly a one-time increase in spending of 5 to 8 percent. This is not an insignificant rise, but it is considerably less than the more than 11 percent annual increase in health care expenditures from 1987 to 1989. It is about as much as the increase in health care spending, *excluding inflation*, in one year to one and a half years.

In global terms, "affordable" can be viewed as the amount the nation thinks it can spend on health care. It can also be considered only as it relates to public expenditures for health care. Finally, it is important to take into account whether the various participants and payers will consider that they can afford the financial obligations they will be required to undertake. The latter view of affordability will involve particularly difficult problems with respect to employers and others who in the past have chosen not to assume financial obligations for health care.

The amount of funds that can be considered "adequate" must be sufficient to pay for the benefits to which the program entitles participants. These funds may come from a number of sources. Both the total amount and the amount from each funding source must be adequate. Costs should be estimated realistically in light of the nature and scope of the benefits offered, the necessity to ensure quality care and reasonable payments for the services of providers. Underfunding, which would result in participants not getting care to which they were entitled, would simply engender suspicion, disillusionment, dissatisfaction, and ultimately opposition to the program.

"Equity" is often in the eye of the beholder, and it will not be easy to get agreement on what constitutes equitable financing. One principle that has had considerable support in the past is that individual payment requirements should be based on ability to pay. Ideally that might mean that the wealthy would pay a higher proportion of their incomes than those not as well-off. Less drastic would be a payment system where people paid the same proportion of their incomes. As previously stated, this is a principle that can be more easily applied to participants in a public program than to those covered privately. Another aspect of equity is that any cost sharing should not be so costly to some in relation to their income or health care condition that it prevents them from getting the care they need.

A favorable impact on the competitiveness of the American economy. This can be considered in two ways — in both the domestic and the international economies. A requirement that all employers bear a fair share of health care costs will eliminate the unfair advantage that employers who do not pay for their employees' health care now have over their competitors who bear such costs. In fact, the payments of the employers who do provide care tend to reflect the health care costs attributable to uninsured employees as well as those of their own workers. Spreading the financial obligation for health care to all employers will enhance competitiveness within the American economy. But if the health care program includes a strong element of cost control, it will also enhance American industry's competitiveness in international markets.

Compatibility with American traditions, principles and institutions. For far-reaching health care reform to be adopted and then made effective, it will have to have broad public understanding and support. It will require federal legislation that will have to pass both Houses of Congress and be signed by the President. This will not happen unless there is a broad consensus that the reform is necessary and will be viable. There must be a clearly defined route from where we are now to the kind of health care system that we seek to achieve. The goals that have been set forth above can be achieved by modifying the current health care system in ways that are compatible with American traditions. Elements such as a public-private program, opportunity for choice and emphasis on quality, affordability and equity are in the American tradition and are compatible with cherished American principles.

It is also in the American tradition that before any new program is adopted, it is subject to much discussion, negotiation and compromise. None of the proposals already offered or to come in the months ahead will be adopted in their original form. In all likelihood, efforts will be made to resolve differences among them and, in the best of circumstances, a refined proposal will eventually come forth that can win broad support. It will be very important for proponents of particular approaches to be willing to compromise so that agreement can be reached. Nevertheless, especially if the compromise involves changes that will limit the scope or effectiveness of the program, it is essential that its supporters not claim more for the program than it can reasonably be expected to achieve. If, when the program is in its initial stages of implementation, people realize that it cannot live up to its promise, it is exceedingly unlikely that the program can succeed.

The nation has an opportunity, perhaps an unprecedented opportunity, to reform the health care system in ways that will greatly enhance its effectiveness and equity and that will assure access to health care that many Americans lack today. This opportunity could pass us by. Therefore, it is most important that we, as a nation, seize it while we can. Organizations like the National Planning Association can make a significant contribution by informing people about the problems that we face in health care and how we can meet them. If there is both broad public understanding of the issues and a political will for action, we can achieve a system that assures affordable quality health care to all Americans.

Bibliography

AFL-CIO. *Bargaining for Access, Quality and Cost.* Washington, D.C., March 1990.

———. *National Health Care - Now Is the Time: The AFL-CIO Campaign for Health Care Reform.* Washington, D.C., 1990.

AFL-CIO Healthcare Committee. *Background on Major Healthcare Reform Options.* Washington, D.C., 1990.

Ball, Robert M. with Thomas N. Bethell. *Because We're All in This Together: The Case for a National Long Term Care Insurance Policy.* Families U.S.A. Foundation. Washington, D.C., 1989.

Burke, Thomas P. and Rita S. Lain. "Trends in Employer-provided Health Care Benefits." *Monthly Labor Review,* February 1991.

Center for the Study of Social Policy. *Kids Count Data Book.* Washington, D.C., 1991.

Digest of National Health Care Use and Expense Indicators. Compiled for the Dunlop Group of Six by the Office of Health Coalitions and Private Sector Initiatives, American Hospital Association. October 1990.

Employee Benefit Research Institute (EBRI). *Features of Employer-Sponsored Health Plans* (EBRI Issue Brief). March 1990.

———. *Uninsured in the United States: The Nonelderly Population without Health Insurance, 1988.* Washington, D.C., September 1990.

———. *Uninsured in the United States: The Nonelderly Population without Health Insurance - Analysis of the March 1990 Current Population Survey.* Washington, D.C., April 1991.

Employee Benefits Management. *Cost Containment, The Health Benefit Challenge of the '90s.* Chicago: Commerce Clearing House, Inc., January 1990.

Evans, Robert G. "Split Vision: Interpreting Cross-Border Differences in Health Spending." *Health Affairs,* Winter 1988.

Fein, Rashi. *Medical Care, Medical Costs: The Search for a Health Insurance Policy.* Harvard University Press, 1986.

Fuchs, Victor R. and James S. Hahn. "How Does Canada Do It? A Comparison of Expenditures for Physicians' Services in the United

States and Canada." *New England Journal of Medicine* (323:884-890), September 27, 1990.

Health Insurance Association of America. *The Health Insurance Industry Strategy for Containing Health Care Costs.* A Report to the Board of Directors. Washington, D.C., February 1990.

Institute of Medicine, Division of Health Care Services. *Medicare — A Strategy for Quality Assurance.* Vol. I. Ed. Kathleen N. Lohr. Washington, D.C.: National Academy Press, 1990.

National Conference of State Legislatures. *Medical Indigency and Uncompensated Health Care Costs.*

Newhouse, Joseph P., Geoffrey Anderson and Leslie L. Roos. "Hospital Spending in the United States and Canada: A Comparison." *Health Affairs,* Winter 1988.

New York State Department of Health. *Universal Health Care: Voices from the State: State Initiatives.* Albany, New York, May 1990.

Reinhardt, Uwe E. *West Germany's Health-Care and Health-Insurance System: Combining Access with Cost Control.* Report prepared for the United States Bipartisan Commission on Comprehensive Health Care, August 30, 1989.

Report of the National Leadership Commission on Health Care. *For the Health of a Nation: A Shared Responsibility.* Washington, D.C., January 1989.

Rivlin, Alice M. and Joshua M. Wiener, with Raymond J. Hanley and Denise A. Spence. *Caring for the Disabled Elderly: Who Will Pay?* Washington, D.C.: Brookings Institution, 1988.

Service Employees International Union, Department of Public Policy. *Labor and Management on a Collision Course Over Health Care.* Washington, D.C., February 1990.

TIAA-CREF. "Health Care Access and Delivery: A Look Ahead." *Research Dialogues,* Number 27, October 1990.

National Planning Association

NPA is an independent, private, nonprofit, nonpolitical organization that carries on research and policy formulation in the public interest. NPA was founded during the Great Depression of the 1930s when conflicts among the major economic groups — business, labor, agriculture — threatened to paralyze national decisionmaking on the critical issues confronting American society. It was dedicated to the task of getting these diverse groups to work together to narrow areas of controversy and broaden areas of agreement as well as to map out specific programs for action in the best traditions of a functioning democracy. Such democratic and decentralized planning, NPA believes, involves the development of effective governmental and private policies and programs not only by official agencies but also through the independent initiative and cooperation of the main private sector groups concerned.

To this end, NPA brings together influential and knowledgeable leaders from business, labor, agriculture, and the applied and academic professions to serve on policy committees. These committees identify emerging problems confronting the nation at home and abroad and seek to develop and agree upon policies and programs for coping with them. The research and writing for these committees are provided by NPA's professional staff and, as required, by outside experts.

In addition, NPA's professional staff undertakes research through its central or "core" program designed to provide data and ideas for policymakers and planners in government and the private sector. These activities include research on national goals and priorities, productivity and economic growth, welfare and dependency problems, employment and human resource needs, and technological change; analyses and forecasts of changing international realities and their implications for U.S. policies; and analyses of important new economic, social and political realities confronting American society.

In developing its staff capabilities, NPA has increasingly emphasized two related qualifications. First is the interdisciplinary knowledge required to understand the complex nature of many real-life problems. Second is the ability to bridge the gap between theoretical or highly technical research and the practical needs of policymakers and planners in government and the private sector.

Through its committees and its core program, NPA addresses a wide range of issues. Not all of the NPA Trustees or committee members are in full agreement with all that is contained in NPA publications unless such endorsement is specifically stated.

81

83

NPA Committee on New American Realities

The Committee on New American Realities — established in 1981 by the National Planning Association — is a private sector group promoting the achievement of a more competitive U.S. economy. Its members are drawn from business, labor, agriculture, and the academic and applied professions. The NAR sponsors open, nonpartisan analysis and discussion of U.S. economic performance to help define common interests and to foster a broad-based consensus out of which effective national policies and private sector initiatives are developed. NAR meetings are designed to encourage frank, informed discussions of issues important to members. NAR formal views and private-public policy recommendations are disseminated in Committee statements and in published research findings.

Work Program

The NAR has identified several major issues that are relevant to the interests of its members:
- U.S. macroeconomic strategies and choices to sustain U.S. competitiveness;
- U.S. workforce preparedness: opportunities for a private-public system of labor market adjustments;
- labor-business relations and the joint responsibility to promote economic growth and employment opportunities.

The Committee's pathbreaking study on *Turbulence in the American Workplace,* published by Oxford University Press in 1991, examines the severe structural changes in the U.S. economy caused by intense global competition and rapid technological advances. This comprehensive work develops a policy agenda for a private-public workforce preparedness system that would enhance the productivity of workers and provide a bulwark against economic hardship. In 1990, NAR published its recommendations on *Preparing for Change: Workforce Excellence in a Turbulent Economy.*

The Committee is completely self-supporting, financed by annual tax-exempt contributions obtained by its members from their organizations.

For further information about NAR's continuing activities, please contact:

James A. Auerbach
NPA Vice President,
and NAR Director

National Planning Association
1424 16th Street, NW, Suite 700
Washington, DC 20036
Tel (202) 265-7685   Fax (202) 797-5516

Members of the NAR

CHARLES R. LEE
Chair;
President and
Chief Operating Officer,
GTE Corporation

MICHAEL A. CALLEN
Vice Chair;
Director and Sector Executive,
Citibank, N.A.

PAUL A. ALLAIRE
Chairman and
Chief Executive Officer,
Xerox Corporation

ELIZABETH E. BAILEY
Visiting Scholar at Yale,
School of Organization &
Management;
Professor of Economics, Industrial
Administration & Public Policy,
Carnegie Mellon University

AL BILIK
President,
Public Employee Department,
AFL-CIO

JAMES B. BOOE
Secretary-Treasurer,
Communications Workers
of America

DENIS BOVIN
Managing Director,
Salomon Brothers

JOHN B. CARON
President,
Caron International

RICHARD W. CORDTZ
Secretary-Treasurer,
Service Employees International
Union, AFL-CIO

JOHN DECONCINI
President,
Bakery, Confectionery
and Tobacco Workers
International Union

JOHN T. DUNLOP
Lamont University
Professor Emeritus,
Economics Department,
Harvard University

JAMES D. EDWARDS
Managing Partner - The Americas,
Arthur Andersen & Co.

DONALD F. EPHLIN
Visiting Senior Fellow,
National Planning Association

MURRAY H. FINLEY
President Emeritus,
Amalgamated Clothing &
Textile Workers' Union;
Chairman of the Advisory
Committee, Amalgamated Bank
of New York

THEODORE GEIGER
Distinguished Research Professor
of Intersocietal Relations,
Georgetown University

ROBERT A. GEORGINE
President,
Building & Construction Trades
Department, AFL-CIO

JACK GOLODNER
President,
Department for Professional
Employees, AFL-CIO

JOSEF E. GRAY
Executive Vice President and
Manager, Human Resources,
Seattle First National Bank

JACK M. GREENBERG
Senior Executive Vice President
and Chief Financial Officer,
McDonald's Corporation

GERALD R. GRINSTEIN
Chairman,
Burlington Northern, Inc.

DALE E. HATHAWAY
Visiting Fellow,
Resources for the Future

R.J. HILDRETH
Managing Director,
Farm Foundation

ROY B. HOWARD
Senior Vice President,
Corporate Human Resources,
BellSouth Corporation

CHARLES S. JOHNSON
Senior Vice President,
Pioneer Hi-Bred
International, Inc.

EDWARD G. JORDAN
Carmel, California

EUGENE J. KEILIN
Senior Partner,
Keilin & Bloom

WILLIAM K. KETCHUM
Vice President of Labor Relations,
AT&T

RICHARD J. KRUIZENGA
Vice President,
Corporate Planning,
Exxon Corporation

JOHN S. REED
Chairman,
Citicorp

ROBERT L. SHAFER
Vice President-Public Affairs
& Government Relations,
Pfizer Inc.

JACK SHEINKMAN
President,
Amalgamated Clothing & Textile
Worker's Union

ROBERT C. STEMPEL
Chairman and Chief Executive
Officer,
General Motors Corporation

PATRICK A. TOOLE
Senior Vice President and
General Manager of Operations,
IBM United States

RICHARD L. TRUMKA
International President,
United Mine Workers of America

BRIAN TURNER
Executive Assistant to
the President,
Industrial Union Department,
AFL-CIO

J.C. TURNER
General President Emeritus,
International Union of
Operating Engineers

Advisors to the Committee

DENNIS J. BLAIR
Executive Assistant to the
Chairman and the President,
GTE Corporation

RICHARD W. HALLOCK
IBM Director of Employee
Relations & Planning,
IBM Corporate Headquarters

Staff

JAMES A. AUERBACH
NAR Director and
NPA Vice President

NPA Publications

Curing U.S. Health Care Ills, by Bert Seidman (104 pp, 1991, $12.00), NAR #6.

Trade Talks with Mexico: A Time for Realism, by Peter Morici (132 pp, 1991, $15.00), CIR #22.

A Time for Action: Ensuring the Stability of the U.S. Financial System, by Robert M. Dunn, Jr., and Richard S. Belous (48 pp, 1991, $5.00), NPA #251.

United Germany and the United States, by Michael A. Freney and Rebecca S. Hartley (196 pp, 1991, $17.50), CIR #21.

The Question of Saving, by Harold Rose (64 pp, 1991, $8.00), BN #38.

Turbulence in the American Workplace, An NAR commissioned study, available from Oxford University Press (270 pp, 1991, $27.95).

Taking Advantage of America's Window of Opportunity, A Statement by the Board of Trustees of the National Planning Association (16 pp, 1990, $2.50), NPA #248.

Creating a Strong Post-Cold War Economy, by Richard S. Belous (40 pp, 1990, $8.00), NPA #247.

Man and His Environment, by Harry G. Johnson, An Occasional Paper (44 pp, 1973, 1990 reprint, $8.00), BN-OP #6.

Transforming the Mexican Economy: The Salinas Sexenio, by Sidney Weintraub (92 pp, 1990, $12.00), CIR #20.

Preparing for Change: Workforce Excellence in a Turbulent Economy, Recommendations of the Committee on New American Realities (32 pp, 1990, $5.00), NAR #5.

Changing Sources of U.S. Economic Growth, 1950-2010: A Chartbook of Trends and Projections, by Nestor E. Terleckyj (76 pp, 1990, $15.00), NPA #244.

The Growth of Regional Trading Blocs in the Global Economy, ed. Richard S. Belous and Rebecca S. Hartley (168 pp, 1990, $15.00), NPA #243.

Continental Divide: The Values and Institutions of the United States and Canada, by Seymour Martin Lipset (326 pp, 1989, $13.00), CAC #59.